# OBSTETRIC
## SURVIVAL

# H A N D B O O K

Yondell Masten, R.N.C., Ph.D., O.G.N.P.

Contributor
Barbara Sagel, R.N., M.S., C.C.R.N.
Critical Care Nurse Specialist
Centura St. Anthony Hospital Central
Denver, Colorado

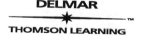

**DELMAR**

**THOMSON LEARNING**

Africa • Australia • Canada • Denmark • Japan • Mexico • New Zealand • Philippines
Puerto Rico • Singapore • Spain • United Kingdom • United States

## NOTICE TO THE READER

COPYRIGHT © 1997 Delmar, a division of Thomson Learning, Inc. The Thomson Learning™ is a trademark used herein under license.

Printed in the United States of America
2 3 4 5 6 7 8 9 10 XXX 03 02 01 00

For more information, contact Delmar, 3 Columbia Circle, PO Box 15015, Albany, NY 12212-0515; or find us on the World Wide Web at http://www.delmar.com

**Library of Congress Cataloging-in-Publication Data**
Masten, Yondell, R.N.C., Ph.D.
The Obstetric Survival Handbook
ISBN: 1-56930-083-6
1. Nursing Handbooks, Manuals
2. Medical Handbooks, Manuals

# TABLE OF CONTENTS

**Introduction** ...................................................1

How to Use This Book ................................... 3

The Mark of a Professional Nurse ................... 4

Standards of Clinical Nursing Practice............ 5

Standards of Professional Performance .......... 6

Care of Women and Newborns ....................... 6

Standards of Care........................................... 7

Standards of Professional Performance ........ 10

**Assessment** ..............................................**19**

The Initial Interview..................................... 21

Admission Patient History ............................ 22

History of Health Habits............................... 29

Prenatal Risk Factors................................... 33

Episodic History .......................................... 37

Subsequent Visit History.............................. 40

Well-Being Assessments............................... 42

Pregnancy Weight Gain and Loss Chart........ 44

Height and Weight Chart............................... 46

Complications of Pregnancy.......................... 47

**Clinical Skills** ...........................................**49**

Estimated Date of Delivery........................... 51

Leopold's Maneuvers.................................... 52

Tips for Performing Maneuvers..................... 53

HIV Pre-Test Counseling .................................................. 54

HIV Post-Test Counseling: Negative ........................... 57

HIV Post-Test Counseling: Positive ........................... 59

Standard Precautions Against AIDS ........................... 61

Fundal Height Measurement ....................................... 65

Bishop's Scale ................................................................. 66

Stages of Labor and Associated Changes .................... 67

Breathing Techniques .................................................... 74

Fetal Monitoring ............................................................ 76

Danger Signs During Labor ......................................... 80

Apgar Scoring System ................................................... 81

Umbilical Cord Care ..................................................... 81

Cardiopulmonary Resuscitation .................................. 82

Neonatal Physical Assessment ..................................... 85

Assessment of Gestational Age .................................... 91

Isolation Procedures ..................................................... 97

Isolation Levels .............................................................. 100

**Teaching Topics** ........................................... **103**

Problems of Pregnancy and Interventions .................. 105

Signs of Labor ................................................................ 112

Pain Management During Labor ................................. 114

The Basic Four Food Pyramid Guide ........................ 116

Recommended Daily Allowances ................................. 119

Recommended Dietary Allowances ............................. 120

Recommended Nutrient Supplementation .................. 129

Food Sources of Nutrients ............................................. 131

Complications of Pregnancy and Treatments ............. 134

Hyperemesis Gravidarum ............................................. 136

Pregnancy-Induced Hypertension ............................... 137

Symptoms of PIH ........................................................... 138

Ectopic Pregnancy ........................................................ 140

The Peurperium .............................................................. 141

Maternal Comfort Measures ....................................... 143

Maternal Self-Care Measures ...................................... 147

Infant Care Measures ................................................... 149

Guidelines for Calling Health Care Provider ............. 150

Adjustment to Parenting Role ..................................... 151

Summary of Methods of Contraception ..................... 152

**Clinical Values and Standards ...................... 165**

Standard Laboratory Values ....................................... 167

Laboratory Findings in Pregnancy ............................. 174

High-Risk Population Prenatal
    Laboratory Screening ............................................... 177

Fetal Well-Being Screening ......................................... 178

Neonatal Well-Being Screening ................................... 178

Screening for Complications of Childbearing ............. 178

Laboratory Values in the Neonatal Period ................. 179

Common Abbreviations ................................................ 184

Measurement Equivalents ............................................ 192

24-Hour Clock .............................................................. 193

# Drug Administration ..................................... 195
Drugs Contraindicated During Breast Feeding.......... 197
Medications During Breast Feeding ........................... 197
Commonly Used Medications Containing Aspirin .... 198
FDA Pregnancy Categories..................................... 199
Commonly Used Medications ................................... 199
Medications Used in Complications ........................... 213
Toxic Chemical Agents............................................ 230
Nursing Interventions for Emergencies...................... 230

# Nursing Care Planning ..................................231
The Nursing Process................................................ 233
The Nursing Process in Action ................................. 234
Guidelines for Therapeutic Communication.............. 236
Barriers to Therapeutic Communication ................... 238
Documentation: The Vital Link to Communication 239
What to Chart.......................................................... 239
How to Chart........................................................... 241
Protecting Yourself Legally....................................... 242
More Guidelines to Prevent Malpractice................... 243

# Professional Network ...................................245
How to Write a Resume............................................ 247
Guidelines to a Successful Job Interview................... 249
Boards of Nursing By State ...................................... 250
State Nurses Associations......................................... 261
Nurses Organizations............................................... 266

Resources for Maternal Care Nurses............................ 269

Professional Organizations ........................................... 273

Public Health Organizations ....................................... 274

Sex Education and Therapy ......................................... 274

Sexually-Transmitted Diseases .................................... 275

**Appendix A** ................................................................**277**

AWHONN Standards & Guidelines
   Table of Contents ..................................................... 279

Selected Obstetric AWHONN Guidelines ................. 281

AWHONN PDMS Phone Number............................. 290

AWHONN On-Line Address ....................................... 290

**Appendix B: Cervical Dilatation**................. **291**

**Index** ......................................................................... **297**

# INTRODUCTION

# INTRODUCTION

How to Use This Book . . . . . . . . . . . . . 3
The Mark of a Professional Nurse . . . . . . . . 4
Standards of Clinical Nursing Practice . . . . . . 5
Standards of Professional Performance . . . . . . 6
Care of Women and Newborns . . . . . . . . . 6
Standards of Care . . . . . . . . . . . . . . 7
Standards of Professional Performance . . . . . . 10

# HOW TO USE THIS BOOK

The *Obstetric Survival Handbook* is a companion to the popular *Nurse's Survival Guide.* This book is not just another spectator manual in nursing written by uninvolved nurses. This is a book that you can really use, especially when confronted with unfamiliar assignments.

This book is about accountability.  By having information readily available, it is hoped that the nurse and the nursing student will increase their accountability in situations where they would otherwise feel uncomfortable. Accountability is the hallmark of nursing care, and nurses are constantly being called upon to fulfill the demands that accountability affords.

This book is not intended to replace a nursing textbook. Instead, it will complement textbooks as an easy-to-grab handbook.  This book presents information that nurses may use frequently but not necessarily memorize. It is a handbook loaded with guidelines, assessment forms, and charts of information.  This book is not intended to offer extensive rationale. When you do not understand the rationale, then is time to research the subject in a comprehensive maternal-child textbook.

## THE MARK OF A PROFESSIONAL NURSE

The basic requirements of a profession are:

- Educational requirements
- Unique knowledge and skills based upon theory
- Service to society
- Autonomy in decision-making and practice
- A code of ethics for practice
- Some degree of status within the role

These requirements are inherent in the foundation of professional nursing. The profession of compassionate caring that Florence Nightingale embraced for nursing is the interpersonal expertise unique to each nurse. These interpersonal skills are intimately interwoven with the professional skills. Never are these interpersonal skills more essential than with obstetric nursing.

Interpersonal skills encompass all the human actions that respect the body, mind and spirit of another person. It is looking at the patient with kindness, listening with empathy, and responding with compassion. A professional nurse offers much more than technical skills, although more and more, technical skills are required.

What do patients want in a nurse? This question has been researched, and it has been found that they want empathy, sensitivity, experience (skills), caring and a sense of confidence, in that order. What they do not want is a nurse who is insensitive, in a hurry, with an air of power. Patients tend to feel uncomfortable with nurses who are unsure of what they are doing.

It is impossible to label the characteristic that makes a nurse professional. That essential quality is elusive, perhaps indescribable. But, when you meet a nurse who has it, you know.

# STANDARDS OF CLINICAL NURSING PRACTICE

The American Nurses' Association sets a standard for nursing that focuses on practice. When nursing care is measured, accountability is also measured by how these standards are concurrently utilized. The ANA Standards of Clinical Nursing Practice are used for measuring accountability in nursing.

The first standards were published in 1973. In 1989, a task force began revising these standards, and these standards were published in 1991. The major change is the emphasis on clinical nursing practice. The standards now address the full scope of practice and are divided into two parts— Standards of Care and Standards of Professional Performance.

## Standards of Care

| | |
|---|---|
| ✳ Assessment | ✳ Diagnosis |
| ✳ Collegiality | ✳ Planning |
| ✳ Implementation | ✳ Evaluation |
| ✳ Quality of care | ✳ Performance appraisal |
| ✳ Education | ✳ Ethics |
| ✳ Collaboration | ✳ Research |
| ✳ Resource utilization | ✳ Outcome identification |

"Standards of Care" describe a competent level of nursing care as demonstrated by the nursing process, involving assessment, nursing diagnosis, outcome identification, planning, implementation, and evaluation. The nursing process encompasses all significant actions taken by nurses in providing care to all clients and forms the foundation of clinical decision-making. Additional nursing responsibilities for all clients (such as providing culturally and ethnically relevant care, maintaining a safe environment, educating clients about their illnesses, treatment, health promotion or self-care activities, and planning for continuity of care) are explained within these standards. Therefore, "Standards of Care" delineate care that is provided to all clients of nursing services.

## STANDARDS OF PROFESSIONAL PERFORMANCE

"Standards of Professional Performance" describe a competent level of behavior in the professional role including activities related to quality of care, performance appraisal, education, collegiality, ethics, collaboration, research, and resource utilization. All nurses are expected to engage in professional role activities appropriate to their education, position and practice setting. While this is no assumption of all of the "Standards of Professional Performance," the scope of nursing involvement in some professional roles is particularly dependent upon the nurse's education, position, and practice environment. Therefore, some standards or measurement criteria identify a broad age of activities that may demonstrate compliance with the standards.

## CARE OF WOMEN AND NEWBORNS

The Association of Women's Health, Obstetric and Neonatal Nurses (AWHONN) publishes the "Standards and Guidelines for Professional Nursing Practice in the Care of Women and Newborns."

# STANDARDS OF CARE

## STANDARD I. Assessment

*The nurse collects the woman's or newborn's health data.*

### Measurement Criteria

1. The priority of data collection is determined by the patient's immediate condition or needs for health maintenance.

2. Pertinent data are collected using appropriate assessment techniques.

3. Data collection involves the patient, significant others, and health care providers, when appropriate.

4. The data collection process is systematic and ongoing.

5. Relevant data are documented in a retrievable form.

## STANDARD II. Diagnosis

*The nurse analyzes the assessment data in determining diagnoses.*

### Measurement Criteria

1. Diagnoses are derived from the assessment data.

2. Diagnoses are validated with the patient, significant others, and health care providers, when possible.

3. Diagnoses are documented in a manner that facilitates the determination of unexpected outcomes and plan of care.

## STANDARD III. Outcome Identification

*The nurse identifies expected outcomes individualized to the woman or newborn.*

### Measurement Criteria

1. Outcome measures are derived from the diagnoses.
2. Outcome measures are documented as measurable goals.
3. Outcome measures are mutually formulated with the patient and healthcare provider when possible.
4. Outcome measures are realistic in relation to the patient's present and potential capabilities.
5. Outcome measures are attainable in relation to resources available to the patient.
6. Outcome measures include a time estimate for attainment.
7. Outcome measures provide direction for continuity of care.

## STANDARD IV. Planning

*The nurse develops a plan of care that prescribes interventions to attain expected outcomes.*

### Measurement Criteria

1. The plan is individualized to the patient's condition or needs.
2. The plan is developed with the patient, significant others, and health care providers, when appropriate.
3. The plan reflects current nursing practice.
4. The plan is documented.
5. The plan provides for continuity of care.

## STANDARD V. Implementation

*The nurse implements the interventions identified in the plan of care.*

### Measurement Criteria

1. Interventions are consistent with the established plan of care.

2. Interventions are consistent with nursing practice that reflects current research and sciences.

3. Interventions may be collaborative and interdependent with other care providers or independent nursing actions.

4. Interventions are implemented in a safe and appropriate manner.

5. Interventions are documented.

## STANDARD VI. Evaluation

*The nurse evaluates the patient's progress toward attainment of outcomes.*

### Measurement Criteria

1. Evaluation is systematic and ongoing.

2. The patient's responses to interventions are documented.

3. The effectiveness of interventions is evaluated in relation to outcomes.

4. Ongoing assessment data are used to revise diagnoses, plan of care, interventions, and outcomes, as needed.

5. Revisions in diagnoses, plan of care  and outcomes are documented.

6. The patient, significant others, and health care providers are involved in the evaluation process, when possible.

## STANDARDS OF PROFESSIONAL PERFORMANCE

### STANDARD I. Quality of Care

*The nurse systematically evaluates the quality and effectiveness of nursing practice.*

#### Measurement Criteria

1. The nurse participates in quality of care activities as appropriate to his or her position, education, and practice environment. Such activities may include:

   - Identification of aspects of care important for quality monitoring.
   - Identification of indicators used to monitor quality and effectiveness of nursing care.
   - Collection of data to monitor quality and effectiveness of nursing care.
   - Analysis of quality data to identify opportunities for improving care.
   - Formulation of recommendations to improve nursing practice or patient outcomes.
   - Implementation of activities to enhance the quality of nursing practice.
   - Participation on interdisciplinary teams that evaluate clinical practice or health services.
   - Development of policies and procedures to improve quality of care.

2. The nurse uses the results of quality of care activities to initiate changes in practice.

3. The nurse uses the results of quality of care activities to initiate changes throughout the health care delivery system, as appropriate.

## STANDARD II. Performance Appraisal

*The nurse evaluates his or her own nursing practice in relation to professional practice standards and relevant statutes and regulations.*

### Measurement Criteria

1. The nurse engages in performance appraisal on a regular basis, identifying areas of strength as well as areas for professional/practice development.

2. The nurse seeks constructive feedback regarding his/her own practice.

3. The nurse takes action to achieve goals identified during performance appraisal.

4. The nurse participates in peer review as appropriate to the practice setting.

## STANDARD III. Education

*The nurse acquires and maintains current knowledge in nursing practice.*

### Measurement Criteria

1. The nurse participates in ongoing educational activities related to clinical knowledge and professional issues.

2. The nurse seeks experiences to maintain clinical skills.

3. The nurse seeks knowledge and skills appropriate to the practice setting.
4. The nurse demonstrates an integration of knowledge and clinical competence through mechanisms defined at his or her practice setting.

## STANDARD IV. Collegiality

*The nurse contributes to the professional development of peers, colleagues, and others.*

### Measurement Criteria

1. The nurse shares knowledge and skill with colleagues and others.
2. The nurse provides peers with constructive feedback regarding their practice.
3. The nurse mentors novice nurses, and those new to the specialty.
4. The nurse contributes to an environment that is conducive to clinical education of nursing students, as appropriate.

## STANDARD V. Ethics

*The nurse's decisions and actions on behalf of patients are determined in an ethical manner.*

### Measurement Criteria

1. The nurse's practice is guided by the *Code for Nurses.*
2. The nurse maintains patient confidentiality.
3. The nurse acts as a patient advocate.

4. The nurse delivers care in a nonjudgmental and non-discriminatory manner that is sensitive to patient diversity.

5. The nurse delivers care in a manner that preserves and protects patient autonomy, dignity, and rights.

6. The nurse seeks available resources to help formulate ethical decisions.

## STANDARD VI. Collaboration

*The nurse collaborates with the patient, significant others and health care providers in providing patient care.*

### Measurement Criteria

1. The nurse communicates with the patient, significant others, and health care providers regarding patient care and nursing's role in the provision of care.

2. The nurse maintains confidentiality consistent with the rules and regulations of state and federal government or the Canadian provincial government.

3. The nurse consults and collaborates with health care providers for patient care, as needed.

4. The nurse makes referrals, including provisions for continuity of care, as needed.

## STANDARD VII. Research

*The nurse uses research findings in practice.*

### Measurement Criteria

1. The nurse uses interventions substantiated by research as appropriate to his/her position, education, and practice environment.

2. The nurse participates in research activities as appropriate to his/her position, education, and practice environment. Such activities may include the following:

   - Identification of clinical problems suitable for nursing research
   - Participation in data collection
   - Participation in a unit, organization, or community research committee or program
   - Sharing of research activities with others
   - Evaluating the clinical significance and application of research findings from related disciplines
   - Conducting research
   - Critiquing research for application to practice
   - Critiquing research findings in the development of policies, procedures, and guidelines for patient care
   - Participating as a member of funding groups, review panels, committees concerned with human subject review, and institutional review boards (IRBs)
   - Evaluating the effect of nursing practice on patient outcomes.

3. The nurse acquires knowledge of the research process and participates in scientific inquiry according to ethical guidelines.

## STANDARD VIII. Resource Utilization

*The nurse considers factors related to safety, effectiveness, and cost in planning and delivering patient care.*

### Measurement Criteria

1. The nurse evaluates factors related to safety, effectiveness, and cost when two or more practice options would result in the same expected patient outcome.

2. The nurse assigns tasks or delegates care based on the needs of the patient and the knowledge and skill of the provider selected.

3. The nurse assists the patient and significant others in identifying and securing appropriate services available to address health needs.

## STANDARD IX. Practice Environment

*The nurse contributes to the environment of care delivery within the practice setting.*

### Measurement Criteria

1. The nurse promotes a safe and therapeutic environment for the recipients and providers of nursing care.

2. The nurse integrates components of the nursing process: assessment, diagnosis, outcome, identification, planning, implementation and evaluation.

3. The nurse individualizes care and sets priorities to address the patient's physical, psychological, educational, and social needs.

4. The nurse articulates the plan of care to other members of the health care team to promote collaborative efforts in achieving outcomes.

5. The nurse documents the integrated components of the nursing process to show responses to interventions.

6. The nurse fosters the development, regular review, and revision of evidenced-based practice guidelines and organizational policies and procedures.

7. The nurse participates in the integration of caring into the practice environment.

## STANDARD X. Accountability

*The nurse is professionally and legally accountable for his/her practice. The professional registered nurse may delegate to and supervise qualified personnel who provide patient care.*

### Measurement Criteria

1. The nurse practices within the scope defined by the state or Canadian provincial practice act and uses standards established by the professional organizations that address the area of practice.

2. The nurse has knowledge of changing professional and ethical issues and practice.

3. The nurse has knowledge of the practice parameters and guidelines of other organizations that focus on the delivery of health care services to women and newborns.

4. The nurse maintains knowledge and clinical skills through a commitment to ongoing professional education and reading and critiquing of the research and professional literature.

5. The nurse collaborates with the multidisciplinary team, when possible.

6. The nurse participates in the development and implementation of practice parameters that may be used as references for health care providers in the orientation of new personnel and students, in activities related to quality assurance, and in guidance of nursing actions in emergency situations.

7. The nurse participates on committees within the practice setting and in periodic peer evaluation and self-evaluation.

8. The nurse maintains certification within the specialty area of practice, when possible, as a mechanism to demonstrate special knowledge.

9. The nurse participates in evaluation of health care outcomes within the practice setting.

10. The nurse participates in activities that foster professional development, such as maintaining membership in professional and specialty organizations.

*References:*

American Nurses Association. (1985). *Code for nurses with interpretive statements.* Washington, DC: Author.

American Nurses Association. (1991). *Standards of Clinical nursing practice.* Washington, DC: Author.

Canadian Nurses Association. (1991). *Code of ethics for nursing.* Ottawa, Ontario: Author.

*From the AWHONN's Standards and Guidelines for Professional Nursing Practice in the Care of Women and Newborns, 5th edition, 1997.*

# ASSESSMENT

# ASSESSMENT

The Initial Interview . . . . . . . . . . . . . . . . . 21

Admission Patient History . . . . . . . . . . . . . . 22

History of Health Habits . . . . . . . . . . . . . . 29

Prenatal Risk Factors . . . . . . . . . . . . . . . 33

Episodic History . . . . . . . . . . . . . . . . . . 37

Subsequent Visit History . . . . . . . . . . . . . . 40

Well-Being Assessments . . . . . . . . . . . . . . 42

Pregnancy Weight Gain and Loss Chart . . . . . . 44

Height and Weight Chart . . . . . . . . . . . . . 46

Complications of Pregnancy . . . . . . . . . . . . 47

## THE INITIAL INTERVIEW

The purpose of the patient interview initially is to gather data, establish rapport and lay a foundation for trust between the patient and the nurse. An expression of warmth and respect by the nurse facilitates this exchange. The nurse must clearly state any expectations and assess the patient's understanding of the communication.

Give the person special attention at the beginning of the interview by calling the patient by name and using appropriate touch.

- Provide for privacy.
- Do not ask one question after another.
- Encourage the patient to talk by using silence.
- A nonjudgmental attitude is essential.
- Avoid long interviews; the patient may get tired or bored.
- Ask only one question at a time to avoid confusion.
- Avoid leading questions that suggest an expected answer.
- Avoid yes or no questions; open-ended ones are usually best.
- Use positive nonverbal communication, such as leaning forward and talking at the same eye level or maintaining eye contact without staring.
- Smile, use light humor when appropriate.
- Do not state opinions or give advice.
- Tell the patient how this information will be used.

- Actively listen to what the patient says and how she says it.
- Be aware of anxiety exhibited as nervous laughing and restlessness.
- Clarify statements when necessary, but avoid confrontation.
- Repeat important points you want the patient to remember.
- Reward the patient with positive comments at the end of the interview.

## ADMISSION PATIENT HISTORY

The admission patient history needs to be taken only once and is useful when making referrals. The background information gathered will be helpful when performing the physical assessment.

### Biographical Data

Name _____

Address and phone _____

Social Security number _____

Age, birthdate, birthplace_____

Sex _____

Ethnicity _____

Marital status _____

Significant other/contact person _____

Occupation and education _____

Religion _____

Stability of living conditions _____

Economic status_____

## Chief Complaint

What specific problem caused you to seek help today?
How long has this been a problem?
(Record as a quote exactly what the patient says)

_____

_____

_____

_____

## Current Pregnancy History

First day of last menstrual period (LMP)_____
Date, results, and type of pregnancy test _____
Symptoms of pregnancy _____
Bleeding and/or cramping since LMP _____
Vaginal discharge_____
Personal risk factors _____
Environmental risk factors_____
Maternal health risk factors _____
Maternal current/past gestational risk factors _____

_____

Maternal feelings regarding pregnancy _____
Gestational age at initiation of prenatal care_____
Prepregnancy weight _____
First day of last normal menstrual period (LNMP), if
LMP was not normal in terms of length of menstrual
cycle, amount of bleeding, and/or duration of menses __
Body mass index _____

## Past Pregnancy History

Number of pregnancies_____

Number of term deliveries _____

Number of preterm deliveries _____

Number of abortions (induced, spontaneous) _____

Number of living children _____

## For Each Pregnancy

Date of delivery _____

Gestational duration _____

Gestational complications _____

Total weight gain_____

Length and type (induced, augmented, spontaneous) of
labor_____

Type of delivery _____

Type of anesthesia _____

Birthweight and gestational age _____

Prenatal, intrapartal, postpartal, neonatal complications

_____

Type of complications_____

Current health of child _____

## Gynecologic History

Age of menarche _____

Length of menstrual cycle _____

Duration and amount of menses _____

History of dysmenorrhea _____

Previous surgery_____

Previous infection _____

Contraceptive history _____
Date of last Pap smear and results _____

## Sexual History

Age at first intercourse _____
Number and health status of sexual partners_____
Number and health status of partner's partners _____
Satisfaction with intercourse _____
Dyspareunia _____

## Current Medical History

General health status _____
Nutritional status_____
Exercise habits _____
Health promotion habits _____
Use of tobacco, alcohol, street drugs_____
Use of over-the-counter drugs_____
Current prescribed medications_____
Drug and other allergies_____
Disease conditions _____
Allergies_____
Weight loss or gain _____

## Past Medical History

Surgeries _____
Injuries_____
Major illnesses _____
Childhood diseases _____
Immunizations _____

Disease conditions _____

Blood transfusions _____

Hospitalizations _____

### Developmental History

Cognitive level _____

Psychological status _____

Interpersonal relationships _____

Coping strategies _____

Personal stressors _____

Nutritional history _____

24-hour diet recall _____

Nutritional problems _____

### Psychological History

How do you feel about being pregnant? _____

Is the father emotionally supportive of you? _____

How are you doing emotionally? _____

Have you ever been depressed? _____

Are you feeling depressed now? _____

How would you rate your quality of life at present on a scale of 1-10? _____

If less than 10, what would it take to make it a 10? What do you wish were different? _____

Have you had any major losses in the last 3 years—jobs, family, friends, moving, abortions, miscarriages? _

_____

Have you ever been in therapy? _____

Have you sustained any significant losses in your life? _

_____

Coping patterns/mechanisms (past and present) _____

_____

## History of Abuse

Is your partner abusive?_____

Have you been hit or knocked down at any time during your pregnancy? _____

If your partner is abusive, how is this abuse exhibited?_

_____

Are you afraid of your partner? _____

Do you think your partner is in control of you and the relationship? _____

Who controls the money?_____

Have you ever been raped? _____

Do you have any abnormal fears or phobias?_____

_____

Have you ever suffered emotional trauma related to elective or spontaneous abortion?_____

## Sociological History

Significant relationships _____

Support system_____

Recent crises/changes at home or work_____

Hours worked per week _____

Work environment:  stress/satisfaction _____

Living environment _____

Economic status_____

Housing _____

Adequate financial resources _____

Perception of financial needs_____

Financial strain of pregnancy _____

Major stressors at home_____

_____

Number of times each partner has been married_____

_____

Number of children of each partner_____

_____

Highest educational degree of each partner _____

_____

Plans for continued education_____

_____

## Cultural History

Language spoken _____

Place of birth _____

If foreign country, time in USA and cultural practices
that should be honored_____

Religious preference and background including rituals
that should be honored (such as fasting) _____

_____

Maternal attitude toward pregnancy _____

Extended family/support system attitude toward pregnancy

_____

Religiously-based health beliefs_____

Religiously-based pregnancy health beliefs _____

Culturally-based health beliefs _____

_____

Culturally-based pregnancy health beliefs _____

_____

Knowledge regarding pregnancy and parenting_____

_____

## Family Medical History

Multiple births _____

Cesarean births_____

Three generation family genogram:

Congenital diseases _____

Congenital anomalies _____

Disease conditions _____

Cause and age of deaths_____

Current health status of living members _____

# HISTORY OF HEALTH HABITS

## Food and Nutrition

### Height, Weight

Body mass index _____

Ideal weight_____

Recent loss or gain in weight_____

Dieting_____

History of eating disorder _____

Fluid intake/day, including kinds of fluids _____

Snack foods_____
History of fasting_____
Vitamins: kind, amount, reason for taking_____

### Sleep
Hours per night_____
Insomnia _____

### Exercise
Kind_____
Amount _____
Frequency _____

### Environmental Hazards
Physical _____
Chemical _____
Biological_____

### Smoking
Packs/day_____
Kind or brand of cigarettes _____
Age started _____
Attempts to quit: number/method _____
Number of other smokers at home _____
Are you thinking of stopping now? _____

### Alcohol
What kind of alcohol (liquor, beer, wine)?_____
When do you drink?_____
How much do you drink? _____

Do you drink to feel good? _____

How old were you when you started drinking? _____

Do you drink with others or alone?_____

How old were you the first time you got drunk? _____

Have you ever had a problem with drinking? _____

Do you think you have a problem with drinking? _____

Does your partner, or other family members, drink? ___

Have you ever been arrested when drinking?_____

Has anyone ever criticized you for drinking?_____

Have you ever needed a drink in the morning?_____

## Drug Use

Do you use drugs for recreational purposes? _____

What kind of drugs do you use?_____

Has doing drugs ever caused you a problem? _____

How old were you when you started using?_____

Do you use marijuana? Cocaine? Heroine?_____

If so, how are these drugs used?_____

Do you shoot IV drugs?_____

How much are you using a week? _____

When do you use drugs? _____

Have you ever smoked crack?_____

Have you ever shared needles? _____

How much are you doing?_____

How much do drugs cost you per week? _____

## Over-The-Counter Drugs

Names _____

Frequency of use_____

Reason for taking medication _____

## Occupational History

Exposure to teratogenic substances _____

_____

Type of work _____

Frequency and duration of rest periods _____

Meal breaks _____

Hours worked per week _____

Shift work (time) _____

## Partner's Current and Past Medical History

Age _____

Ethnicity _____

Occupation _____

Educational level _____

Blood type and Rh factor _____

Disease conditions _____

Use of tobacco, alcohol, street drugs_____

Genetic conditions _____

Perception of the pregnancy _____

Lifestyle habits _____

## Partner's Family Medical History

Disease conditions _____

Congenital diseases _____

Congenital anomalies _____

Genetic disorders _____

Lifestyle habits _____

# PRENATAL RISK FACTORS

There are certain factors that are associated with increased morbidity and mortality of mothers and infants. These factors should be carefully monitored if assessed during the initial interviews:

**Maternal Characteristics:**

- Age: under 16 or over 35
- Ambivalence toward pregnancy
- Low socio-economic group
- Not married
- Family conflict
- 20% overweight or underweight: inadequate nutrition
- Multiparity > 3
- Smoking ≥ 1 pack per day
- Addicting drugs/alcohol

**Obstetric History**

- More than one abortion
- Gravidity over 8
- Stillbirth
- Neonatal death
- Infant less than 2500 g
- Infant over 4,000 g

- Infant with major disease
- Preeclampsia or eclampsia
- Difficult deliveries
- Rh sensitization
- Genital tract anomaly
- Ovarian masses

**Medical Problems**

- Hypertension: renal
- Heart disease
- Anemia
- Disease: diabetes mellitus
- Endocrine disorder
- Sickle cell disease
- Pulmonary disease

# INITIAL PRENATAL LAB ASSESSMENT

- CBC, type, Rh
- General antibody screen
- Sickle cell screen for black mother
- Pap smear
- Rubella titer
- Urine culture and sensitivity
- Coomb's for Rh negative mother

# ASSESSMENT RELATED TO GENETIC COUNSELING

Family history of a genetic disorder _____

Fetal anomalies detected by ultrasound _____

Pregnancy at age 35 or older_____

Abnormal maternal serum alpha-fetoprotein screen ____

Birth defects in other children: single anomalies, multiple defect patterns _____

History of metabolic disorders in family_____

Mental retardation or developmental delay in any other children in family_____

Chronic neurologic or neuromuscular childhood disorder

_____

Short stature or dysmorphic features_____

_____

Ambiguous genitalia or abnormal sexual development _

_____

Carrier status for a genetic disease in specific populations

_____

Infertility, sterility, multiple pregnancy losses, or stillbirth

_____

Exposure to potentially mutagenic or teratogenic agents

_____

Genetic risk due to consanguinity _____

Adult-onset disability of genetic origin _____

Behavioral disorders of genetic origin _____

Cancer, heart disease, and other common conditions
with a genetic component_____

## NUTRITIONAL ASSESSMENT

Diet dramatically affects a person's state of health. To
assess a patient's nutritional status, first record the typical 24-hour intake, then assess eating habits on a
weekly basis. After completing the assessment, you can
evaluate the adequacy of the diet according to the
guidelines established by the basic food groups.

Nutrition for the pregnant woman consists of eating a
well-balanced diet based on the Food Pyramid. Specific needs for pregnancy and lactation are noted in additional requirements listed in the RDA.

Name _____

Age/Sex _____

Marital status _____

Occupation _____

BMI _____

Recent weight loss _____

Medical diagnosis _____

Food restrictions (medical or religious)_____

Ethnic and economic background _____

Problems with eating, general conditions of teeth_____

Food allergies_____

Food preferences _____

Daily nutritional supplements_____

Patient complaints (weakness, indigestion, skin problems)

_____

Elimination habits _____

Use of laxatives _____

# EPISODIC HISTORY

Episodic history assessments are made at each prenatal visit. The episodic history includes a summary of physical and emotional problems and complaints since the previous prenatal visit. Specific questions can be asked based on expected needs of each trimester. The following is a sample list by trimester:

## FIRST TRIMESTER

### Discomforts

- Breast changes
- Fatigue
- Nausea and/or vomiting
- Nasal stuffiness and/or epistaxis

- Family dynamics
- Gingivitis
- Leukorrhea

- Psychosocial responses

### Self-Care

- Exercise
- Rest and relaxation

- Nutrition

**Warning or Danger Signs**

- Bleeding
- Chills and fever
- Persistent, severe vomiting
- Burning on urination
- Cramping diarrhea

## SECOND TRIMESTER

### Discomforts

- Faintness
- Gastrointestinal distress
- Neuromuscular distress
- Psychosocial responses
- Skin changes
- Family dynamics
- Gingivitis
- Palpitations
- Skeletal distress
- Varicosities

### Self-Care

- Exercise
- Rest and relaxation
- Nutrition
- Sexuality

### Warning or Danger Signs

- Bleeding
- Chills and fever
- Decreased or absent fetal movements
- Ruptured membranes
- Burning on urination
- Diarrhea
- Persistent, severe vomiting

## THIRD TRIMESTER

### Discomforts

- Ankle edema
- False labor
- Fatigue
- Insomnia
- Perineal pressure
- Psychosocial responses
- Heartburn

- Dizziness
- Family dynamics
- Gingivitis
- Leg cramps
- Shortness of breath
- Urinary frequency

- Constipation

### Self-Care

- Baby preparation
- Labor preparation
- Rest and relaxation

- Exercise
- Nutrition
- Sexuality

### Warning or Danger Signs

- Bleeding
- Chills and fever
- Epigastric pain
- Preterm labor
- Severe headache
- Decreased or absent fetal movement
- Oliguria

- Burning on urination
- Diarrhea
- Generalized edema
- Rupture of membranes
- Visual disturbances
- Edema (face, hands, legs)

**Do you have any concerns regarding:**

Sexual activity _____

Fetal movement _____

Weight gain _____

Nutritional status _____

Estimated date of delivery (EDD) _____

**Are you taking any:**

Prescribed medications _____

Over-the-counter medications _____

Laxatives or enemas _____

Nutritional supplements _____

Vitamins and minerals _____

Alcohol beverages _____

Illicit drugs _____

Are you smoking cigarettes? _____

**How are you feeling emotionally:**

Support system_____

Abusive behavior _____

Getting enough rest_____

## SUBSEQUENT VISIT HISTORY

### Chief Complaint

What specific problem caused you to seek help today?

_____

How long has this been a problem?_____

(Record as a quote exactly what the patient says)

_____

_____

_____

## Detailed History of Illness

What: What were you doing at the time the problem occurred?

When: When did it begin (date, time of day)?

How: Was it a recurring or sudden onset? Severity?

Why: Any precipitating events that occurred?

Symptoms of gestational complication _____

_____

Symptoms of labor _____

Frequency and duration of contractions _____

Location of discomfort_____

Quality of fetal movement _____

Status of amniotic membranes _____

Presence and character of vaginal discharge_____

## Pregnancy History for Each Trimester

Bleeding and/or cramping since LMP/last prenatal visit

_____

Vaginal discharge_____

Personal risk factors _____

Environmental risk factors_____

Maternal health risk factors _____

Maternal current/past gestational risk factors _____

Maternal feelings regarding pregnancy _____

Developmental tasks of pregnancy activities _____

# WELL-BEING ASSESSMENTS

Well-being assessments of the mother and fetus involve physical assessment, laboratory tests, and fetal growth data collection. The purpose is to document pregnancy growth and development and to identify potential problems early. Prenatal visits for low-risk clients usually occur every 4 weeks until 32 weeks, every 2 weeks from 32-36 weeks and weekly from 36 weeks gestation to birth. High-risk clients are usually assessed more often. The following assessments are made during each prenatal visit:

**Physical Assessment:**

- Maternal weight gain
- Maternal vital signs
- Fetoscope auscultation from 19 or 20 weeks to birth
- Fetal heart rate (120-160 bpm)
- CVA tenderness
- Edema
- Doppler auscultation from 10 or 12 weeks to 20 weeks
- Homan's sign

## Laboratory Tests:

- Hemoglobin and hematocrit (at 28 weeks)
- Glucose screen at 24-28 weeks
- Urinalysis (each visit)

## Fetal Growth and Development:

- Maternal serum alpha-fetoprotein (at 15-18 weeks)
- Fetal presentation (from 32 weeks to birth)
- Fetal movement (maternal report and examiner palpation)
- Quickening (date of maternal perception of first movement)
- Fundal height (at each visit)

## Pregnancy Weight Gain

The graph plots weight gain by prenatal visit with the pounds of weight gain on the vertical left axis from -8 up to 50 pounds with zero being the prepregnancy weight; the horizontal axis is 0 to 44 weeks gestation.

Recommended weight gain is based on body mass index (BMI) with 1-3 pounds weight gain in the first trimester and the remainder for the second and third trimesters based on the BMI (Institute of Medicine, 1990):

Low BMI (< 19.8 ) = 28-40 lbs (1-1.5 lbs/wk)

Normal BMI (19.8 - 26.0) = 25-35 lbs (0.9-1.3 lbs/wk)

High BMI (26.0 - 29.0) = 15.25 lbs (0.5 lbs/wk)

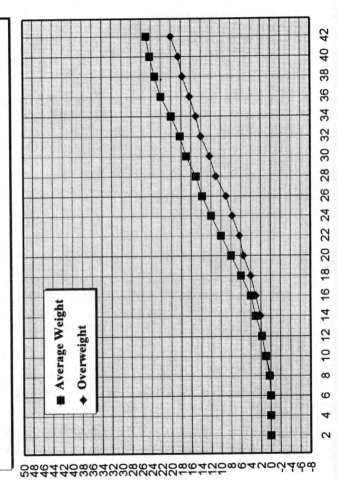

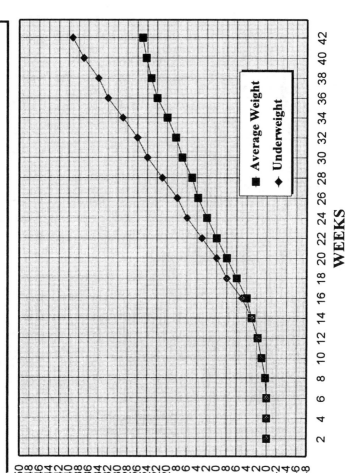

# AVERAGE & UNDERWEIGHT

## Pregnancy Weight Gain and Loss Chart

POUNDS

WEEKS

■ Average Weight
◆ Underweight

# HEIGHT AND WEIGHT CHART

## Metropolitan Life Insurance Company

In 1983 the Metropolitan Life Insurance Company devised a height-weight scale that has become a standard.

### WOMEN

| HEIGHT | | FRAME | | |
| --- | --- | --- | --- | --- |
| Ft. | In. | Small | Medium | Large |
| 4 | 10 | 102-111 | 109-121 | 118-131 |
| 4 | 11 | 103-113 | 111-123 | 120-134 |
| 5 | 0 | 104-115 | 113-126 | 122-137 |
| 5 | 1 | 106-118 | 115-129 | 125-140 |
| 5 | 2 | 108-121 | 118-132 | 128-143 |
| 5 | 3 | 111-124 | 121-135 | 131-147 |
| 5 | 4 | 114-127 | 124-138 | 134-151 |
| 5 | 5 | 117-130 | 127-141 | 137-155 |
| 5 | 6 | 120-133 | 130-144 | 140-159 |
| 5 | 7 | 123-136 | 133-147 | 143-163 |
| 5 | 8 | 126-139 | 136-150 | 146-167 |
| 5 | 9 | 129-142 | 139-153 | 149-170 |
| 5 | 10 | 132-145 | 142-156 | 152-173 |
| 5 | 11 | 135-148 | 145-159 | 155-176 |
| 6 | 0 | 138-151 | 148-162 | 158-179 |

# ASSESSING COMPLICATIONS OF PREGNANCY

- Bleeding anytime, but especially after 20 weeks
- Nutrition
- Hydramnios
- Hypertension
- Rh-negative mother
- Viral infections
- Bacterial infections
- Postmaturity
- Anemia
- PIH
- Spontaneous PROM

- Premature rupture of membranes
- No prenatal care
- Excessive weight loss
- Hyperglycemia
- Exposure to teratogens
- Syphilis
- HIV infected
- Abnormal presentation
- Abruptio placenta
- Placenta previa

# CLINICAL SKILLS

# CLINICAL SKILLS

Estimated Date of Delivery . . . . . . . . . . . . . 51
Leopold's Maneuvers . . . . . . . . . . . . . . . . 52
Tips for Performing Maneuvers . . . . . . . . . . 53
HIV Pre-Test Counseling . . . . . . . . . . . . . 54
HIV Post-Test Counseling: Negative . . . . . . . . 57
HIV Post-Test Counseling: Positive . . . . . . . . 59
Standard Precautions Against AIDS . . . . . . . . 61
Fundal Height Measurement . . . . . . . . . . . . 65
Bishop's Scale . . . . . . . . . . . . . . . . . . . 66
Stages of Labor and Associated Changes . . . . . . 67
Breathing Techniques . . . . . . . . . . . . . . . 74
Fetal Monitoring . . . . . . . . . . . . . . . . . . 76
Danger Signs During Labor . . . . . . . . . . . . 80
Apgar Scoring System . . . . . . . . . . . . . . . 81
Umbilical Cord Care . . . . . . . . . . . . . . . . 81
Cardiopulmonary Resuscitation . . . . . . . . . . 82
Neonatal Physical Assessment . . . . . . . . . . . 85
Assessment of Gestational Age . . . . . . . . . . . 91
Isolation Procedures . . . . . . . . . . . . . . . . 97
Isolation Levels . . . . . . . . . . . . . . . . . . . 100

## ESTIMATED DATE OF DELIVERY

Nägele's rule uses the first day of the last menstrual period (LMP) or the first day of the last normal menstrual period (LNMP) if the last menstrual period was
abnormal in terms of amount or duration of menses.
The EDD determined by Nägele's Rule adds 7 days to
the first day of the LMP, subtracts 3 months from the
month of the LMP, and adds 1 year to the year of the
LMP. The calculated EDD is then considered correct
within 2 weeks. An example would be a client with the
first day of her LMP being July 4, 1998. The calculation would be the following:

|      | Month | Day | Year |
|------|-------|-----|------|
| LMP  | 7     | 4   | 1998 |
| EDD  | -3    | +7  | +1   |
|      | 4     | 11  | 1999 |

Thus, the EDD would be April 11, 1999, and birth
could be expected within 2 weeks before or 2 weeks
after April 11. If the uterine size is approximately the
same as the calculated weeks of gestation, then the data
indicate uterine size and EDD date consistency (abbrevi-
ated as size-date consistency or S=D)

# LEOPOLD'S MANEUVERS

Leopold's maneuvers are four maneuvers implemented to assess fetal position by manually palpating the abdomen. This assessment is used to identify fetal presentation, lie, presenting part, attitude, degree of descent, an estimate of the size, and number of fetuses.

* Determine lie: longitudinal or transverse
* Determine location of the head, back, buttocks
* Determine the presenting part
* Determine engagement of the presenting part
* Size of fetus compared to gestational age
* Determine if more than one fetus is present
* Determine PMI for fetus
* Auscultate FHR
* Determine if fundal height is congruent with gestational age

**First maneuver**

* Patient in supine position with knees slightly flexed
* Put towel under head and right hip
* With both hands, palpate upper abdomen and fundus
* Assess size, shape, movement and firmness of the part
* Head is firm and moveable, breech is soft, less mobile

**Second maneuver**

&ast; With both hands moving down, identify the back

&ast; Note whether back is on left or right side of abdomen

**Third maneuver**

&ast; With the right hand over the symphysis pubis, identify the presenting part by grasping the lower abdomen with thumb and fingers

&ast; Assess whether the presenting part is engaged in the pelvis (if the head is engaged it will not be moveable)

**Fourth maneuver**

&ast; The nurse alters position by turning toward the patient's feet

&ast; With both hands, assess the descent of the presenting part by locating the cephalic prominence or brow

&ast; When the brow is on the same side as the back, the head is extended.  When the brow is on the same side as the small parts, the head will be flexed and the vertex presenting

## TIPS FOR PERFORMING MANEUVERS

&ast; Tell the patient where the fetal heartbeat is found and allow her to listen

&ast; Tell the patient what is assessed:  where the head, the back and buttocks are located.

&ast; Instruct to void before procedure to prevent discomfort.

# HIV PRETEST COUNSELING

## PRE-TEST COUNSELING

1. Assist patient in evaluating risk.

   *Since 1983 have you:*

   Had sex without a condom?

   Used IV drugs? Shared needles?

   Had a blood transfusion of any kind?

   Had a job in which you were exposed to blood, such as with a needle stick?

   Been in any country where HIV is epidemic?

   Had or been exposed to a sexually transmitted disease?

   Had sex with anyone who has been in jail or prison?

2. The pros and cons of testing:

   - If results negative: emotional relief from fear, can take steps to protect self in future

   - If results positive:

     - Able to take steps to decrease symptoms of AIDS

     - Prophylactic medications can "buy time" for curative medicines to be discovered

     - Can take steps to prevent infection of others

     - Can help with personal decision-making in other ways. For example, the test results could help a person decide whether or not to have a baby.

**Disadvantages of positive test**

*Emotional trauma of:*
- Knowing AIDS is always fatal
- Living with uncertainty
- Being known as an infected person and/or person with AIDS with potential for social isolation, harassment
- Recognizing that the disease causes physical pain
- Knowing that personal relationships may be threatened
- Knowing that employment may be threatened
- Knowing potential for transmission to baby if pregnancy occurs
- Fear of infecting others if lifestyle changes not made
- May perpetuate risk behaviors

3. Acknowledge that decision to be tested is difficult, that recognition of risk for a life-threatening illness is involved.

4. Describe procedure:
- Blood draw
- Advise of time period required to obtain results
- Explain that positive results are confirmed with a second test, usually another kind of test
- Explain reasons for requiring test results to be given in person.

5. Discuss the reliability of the test. ELISA is 99% sensitive and specific.

6. Explain the meaning of a negative test.
   - Not exposed to HIV
   - Lag time for development of antibody (6 to 52 weeks)
   - Possible need to be retested.

7. Explain the meaning of a positive test. The HIV positive person is infected and is infectious but does not have AIDS.

8. Explain the differences between anonymous and confidential testing. (Confidential testing restricts test results to the medical file.)

9. Ask patient if more information or time is needed to make a decision.

10. Review ways to avoid exposure.

11. Explain that help will be given to arrange counseling and medical evaluation if test results are positive.

12. Ask how she generally deals with stress/crisis and how she thinks she might deal with learning she is HIV positive.

13. Make an appointment for a follow-up meeting to discuss test results. Discuss the potential for stress/anxiety during this period.

# HIV POST-TEST COUNSELING: NEGATIVE RESULTS

Inform that result is negative. Show client lab result form:

1. Review what a negative test means:
   - The body showed no signs of HIV.
   - If exposure has been recent *(within the last 6 months)* the body may not yet show signs of infection. Therefore, repeat test in 6 months.

2. Explore client's response to negative test result:
   - Determine if there is ongoing risk of exposure
   - Review modes of transmission:
   - Sexual contact
   - Blood/blood product ingestion as with sharing needles
   - Perinatal transmission

3. Provide new information as appropriate about:
   - Safer sex
   - Safer use of drugs

4. Instruct on current selection and application of condoms:
   - Explore feeling about their use.
   - "Have you ever used a condom?"
   - "What was your experience with using them/How do you feel about them?"
   - "Have you ever talked about condoms with your  partner?"

- Demonstrate proper use using a model and encouraging client to touch the condom. Be playful; talk about new ways to make love.

- Explore which condoms might be best for this client.

- Discuss condom lubrication, price, and community resources for free condoms.

- Conduct strategy session that includes a discussion of ways to negotiate with partner for safer sex behaviors.

- Inquire about possible need for partner to come in for counseling/testing.

- Encourage commitment to staying negative.

- Emphasize the need for ongoing testing in association with at-risk behavior.

- Give HIV literature if acceptable to client and appropriate reading level literature is available. (Remember that half of US adults read at or below the 9th grade level and most health education materials are written above the 9th grade level. This information is cited in a useful book titled, *Teaching Patients with Low Literacy Skill* by Cecilia Dosk and Leonard Dosk. It is published by Lippincott.)

# HIV POST-TEST COUNSELING
## POSITIVE RESULT

1.  Make sure the room is private and quiet. Arrange for no interruptions; allow plenty of time. The patient may remember little of what is said. Be patient. Be prepared for shock, denial, anger, confusion, anxiety. Consider the advantages of having two counselors present to provide support.

2.  Inform that test is positive. Hand the patient the lab report so that the results are seen.

3.  Determine the patient's understanding of what a positive test means.

4.  Review the correct meaning of the antibody test as needed
    - Infection with HIV
    - Lifelong infection until treatment/cure discovered
    - At-risk status for AIDS

5.  Review the reliability of the test, if appropriate.

6.  Acknowledge the reasonableness of fear of suffering or dying or repeated losses (physical strength, mental acuity, sexual freedom, self-sufficiency and possibly family, lovers, friends, a job). Do not minimize the gravity of the patient's situation. Do not attempt to assess time frame for development of AIDS.

7.  Discuss patient's support systems within own social network and/or support groups. Make a referral to a support group if appropriate.

8. Explain spectrum of disease if patient seems able/ready to hear. Speak with realistic optimism. Avoid use of the word "victim."

9. Emphasize the importance of a medical evaluation as soon as possible so that a baseline evaluation can be made and prophylactic medication started. Emphasize the importance of a health care provider who has experience with PWAs. Make referral if possible.

10. Assess possibility of pregnancy.

11. If in the childbearing years and not using birth control and/or desirous of pregnancy, encourage to postpone pregnancy until a knowledgeable decision can be made.

12. Begin process of assessing patient's willingness to notify contacts. If the patient is ready to do this, help her plan how it will be done. Key points include a private setting, anticipation of anger/blame, need for testing, and importance of safer sex/safer use.

13. Encourage the patient to think a while before deciding whom else to tell. Rehearse ways to tell others if appropriate.

14. Discuss advisability of testing for potentially infected family members.

15. Emphasize the importance of attention to good health habits including avoiding alcohol, cigarettes, marijuana, and drugs as well as the positive benefits of sleep and good food.

16. Stress the importance of keeping insurance policies up-to-date.

17. Discuss the continuing importance of following safer sex and safer use guidelines to avoid infecting others, to minimize chances for repeated exposure to the virus, and to avoid exposure to other STDs with consequent strain on the immune system.

18. Remind not to donate blood, plasma or body organs. Do not breast feed. Do not share toothbrushes, safety razors or other items that could have blood on them.

19. If appropriate, discuss need for/possible consequences of sharing results with sexual partners, relatives, friends, school, health care providers.

20. Offer literature if deemed appropriate. Be sure that any material given is at an appropriate reading level. Explore with the patient what might happen if the material were to be found by others.

22. Evaluate the potential for suicide.

23. Give phone numbers or office callback and AIDS crisis or information hot lines.

24. Schedule a follow-up counseling appointment within a few days.

## STANDARD PRECAUTIONS AGAINST AIDS

Because the potential for infectivity of any client's blood and body fluids cannot be known, blood and body fluid and substance precautions recommended by the Center for Disease Control and Prevention (CDC) should be adhered to for all clients for all blood and body fluid specimens/contact. These precautions, called "Standard Precautions," should be followed regardless of any lack of evidence of the client's infection status. Routinely use barrier protection to prevent skin and mucous membrane contamination with the following:

a.   secretions and excretions, except sweat, regardless of whether or not they contain visible blood;

b.   body fluids of all clients and client specimens;

c.   nonintact skin; and

d.   mucous membranes.

In addition, health care professionals who have exudative lesions or weeping dermatitis should refrain from all direct client care and from handling client care equipment until the condition is resolved.

## Hand Washing

Frequent handwashing is essential for protection of the client and the care provider. The following are minimal incidences for careful handwashing:

a.   Wash hands after touching blood, body fluids, secretions, excretions, and contaminated items, whether or not gloves are worn. Wash hands immediately after gloves are removed, between client contacts, and when otherwise indicated to avoid transfer of microorganisms to other clients or environments. It may be necessary to wash hands between tasks and procedures on the same client to prevent cross-contamination of different body sites.

b.   Use a plain (nonantimicrobial) soap for routine hand washing.

c.   Use an antimicrobial agent or waterless antiseptic agent for specific circumstances (e.g., control of outbreaks or hyperendemic infections) as defined by the infection control program.

### Gloves

Wear gloves (clean, nonsterile, completely intact gloves [no open fingers/fingertips] are adequate) when touching blood, body fluids, secretions, excretions, and contaminated items, and when performing venipuncture, arterial puncture, skin puncture, and other vascular access procedures. Put on clean gloves just before touching mucous membranes and nonintact skin. Change gloves between tasks and procedures on the same client after contact with material that may contain a high concentration of microorganisms. Remove gloves promptly after use, before touching noncontaminated items and environmental surfaces, and before going to another client. Wash hands immediately to avoid transfer of microorganisms to other clients or environments.

### Mask, Eye Protection, Face Shield

Wear a mask and eye protection or a face shield to protect mucous membranes of the eyes, nose, and mouth during procedures and client care activities that are likely to generate splashes or sprays of blood, body fluids, secretions, and excretions.

### Gown

Wear a gown (a clean, nonsterile gown is adequate) to protect skin and prevent soiling of clothing during procedures and client care activities that are likely to generate splashes or sprays of blood, body fluids, secretions, or excretions or cause soiling of clothing. Select a gown that is appropriate for the activity and amount of fluid likely to be encountered. Remove soiled gown as promptly as possible and wash hands to avoid transfer of microorganisms to other clients or environments.

## Patient Care Equipment

Handle used client care equipment soiled with blood, body fluids, secretions, and excretions in a manner that prevents skin and mucous membrane exposures, contamination of clothing, and transfer of microorganisms to other clients and environments. Ensure that reusable equipment is not used for the care of another client until it has been appropriately cleaned and reprocessed and single use items are properly discarded.

## Environmental Control

Ensure that the hospital/institution/agency has adequate procedures for routine care, cleaning, and disinfection of environmental surfaces, beds, bedrails, bedside equipment, exam tables, and other frequently touched surfaces and that these procedures are being followed.

## Linen

Handle, transport, and process used linen soiled with blood, body fluids, secretions, and excretions in a manner that prevents skin and mucous membrane exposures and contamination of clothing and avoids transfer of microorganisms to other clients and environments.

## Occupational Health and Blood-Borne Pathogens

a.  Take care to prevent injuries when using needles, scalpels, and other sharp instruments or devices; when handling sharp instruments after procedures; when cleaning used instruments; and when disposing of used needles. Never recap used needles or otherwise manipulate them with both hands or any other technique that involves directing the point of the needle toward any part of the body; rather, use either a one-handed scoop technique or a mechanical device designed for holding the nee-

dle sheath. Do not remove used needles from disposable syringes by hand; and do not bend, break, or otherwise manipulate used needles by hand.
Place used disposable syringes and needles, scalpel blades, and other sharp items in appropriate puncture-resistant containers located as close as practical to the area in which the items were used.
Place reusable syringes and needles in a puncture-resistant container for transport to the reprocessing area.

b.  Use mouthpieces, resuscitation bags, or other ventilation devices as an alternative to mouth-to-mouth resuscitation methods in areas where the need for resuscitation is predictable.

**Patient Placement**

Place a client who contaminates the environment or who does not (or cannot be expected to) assist in maintaining appropriate hygiene or environmental control in a private room.  If a private room is not available, consult infection control professionals regarding client placement or other alternatives.

*The above Standard Precautions can be obtained in its entirety from the CDC.*

## FUNDAL HEIGHT MEASUREMENT

* Use nonstretchable tape measure.

* Measure from notch of symphysis pubis to top of the fundus.

* Be careful not to tip back the corpus.

* To determine duration of pregnancy in weeks, use McDonald's rule (during the second and third

trimester): Height of fundus in cm x 8/7 = weeks of pregnancy.

## BISHOP'S SCALE

Bishop's scale for assessing women for induction of labor:

| Score | 0 | 1 | 2 | 3 |
|---|---|---|---|---|
| Dilatation (cm) | 0 | 1-2 | 3-4 | 5-6 |
| Effacement (%) | 0-30 | 40-50 | 60-70 | 80 |
| Station (cm) | -3 | -2 | -1 | +1 |
| Cervical consistency | Firm | Medium | Soft | |
| Fetal position | Posterior | Midline | Anterior | |

**Parous woman can be induced at score of 5; nulliparous woman at score of 7.

| STAGES OF LABOR AND ASSOCIATED CHANGES | |
| --- | --- |
| **STAGE I (LATENT PHASE)** | **CHANGES** **8 1/2 h** |
| Mild, better coordinated contractions (manually or electronically monitored) | Contractions 5-30 min apart, lasting 10-30 sec |
| Cervical dilatation and effacement. Sterile vaginal exam unless bleeding or ruptured membranes present | Dilatation 0-3 cm, complete effacement in primigravida, effacement with dilatation in multigravida |
| Station (measured above or below ischial spines) | Degree of descent 0-2 cm with primigravida experiencing slower rate with little or no descent |
| Mucous plug | Pinkish or brownish mucus vaginal secretions |
| Ruptured membranes | Positive Fern Test; positive nitrazine paper test (blue color) |

| STAGES OF LABOR AND ASSOCIATED CHANGES | |
|---|---|
| Position and presentation of fetus (performing Leopold's maneuver) | Position may be left or right occiput anterior or posterior (LOA, ROA, LOP, ROP); left or right sacrum anterior or posterior (LSA, RSA, LSP, RSP); or other; presentation may be vertex, breech, shoulder |
| Fetal heart tones | Between 120-160 bpm heard below umbilicus for vertex presentation or above umbilicus for breech presentation; increases during fetal movement and possibly uterine contractions |
| Pulse and blood pressure | Remains at baseline levels between uterine contractions |
| **Stage I Labor (Active Phase)** | **Changes 5-6 h primigravida, as little as 2 h multigravida** |
| Moderate, regular fundal dominant contractions | Contractions 2-3 min apart, lasting 45-60 seconds |

| STAGES OF LABOR AND ASSOCIATED CHANGES ||
| --- | --- |
| Cervical dilatation, Friedman graph | Dilatation 4-8 cm, usually 1.2 cm/hr in primigravida, 1.5 cm/hr in multigravida, Friedman graph used to correlate dilatation with fetal descent |
| Station (below ischial spines) | Descent into midpelvis 0-2, at least 1 cm/hr in primigravida, 2 cm/hr in multigravida |
| Vaginal secretions | Moderate to large amounts of bloody mucus, some amniotic fluid if membranes have ruptured |
| Fetal heart tones between contractions | Between 120-160 bpm heard just below umbilicus depending on fetal position with rate responding to contractions and fetal movement |
| Vital signs | Usually at baseline levels but hypotension may occur as a result of regional block or supine hypotension |

| STAGES OF LABOR AND ASSOCIATED CHANGES ||
|---|---|
| **Stage I Labor (Transition Phase)** | **Changes 2 hours in primigravida; 1 hour in multigravida** |
| Strong contractions | Contractions 1½-2 min apart, lasting 60-90 sec |
| Cervical dilatation, urge to push | Dilatation 8-10 cm, with pushing discouraged until cervix is completely dilated |
| Station and effacement | Station of +1 to +3 |
| Vaginal secretions | Increased amounts bloody mucus |
| Fetal heart tones between or after each contraction | Between 120-160 bpm heard slightly above symphysis pubis, rate changes if uterine circulation impaired or if fetal head is compressed |
| Vital signs in between contractions | Slight elevation in pulse and respirations with panting, increased bpm of 10 mmHg over baseline |

## STAGES OF LABOR AND ASSOCIATED CHANGES

| Stage II Labor (Expulsion of Fetus) | Changes 1 hour in primigravida; 15 minutes in multipara |
|---|---|
| Strong contractions | Contractions 2-3 minutes apart, lasting 60-90 seconds |
| Cervical dilatation and effacement | Dilatation 10 cm with complete effacement |
| Station and fetal position | Station reaching +4 as head reaches perineal floor |
| Vaginal secretions | Copious bloody mucus and increased amniotic fluid expelled during contractions |
| Crowning with pushing | Perineal bulging, flattening as fetus descends with head visible |
| Fetal heart tones after each contraction | Between 120-160 bpm with variations of 6-10 bpm, bradycardia may occur during contractions |
| Vital signs between contractions | Increased 5-10 mmHg systolic increase in BP |

| STAGES OF LABOR AND ASSOCIATED CHANGES ||
|---|---|
| Birth of infant, position and presentation | Episiotomy may be done to facilitate birth, prevent tearing; vacuum extraction may be used if stage is prolonged or pushing is inhibited; baby's body will rotate following expulsion of the head, and rest of body is expelled; cord is cut and infant is evaluated by APGAR and placed in warm bassinet |
| **Stage III (Expulsion of placenta)** | **5-15 minutes after birth or after 1st or 2nd contraction as placenta separation takes place** |
| Contractions, height and shape of uterus | Fundus of uterus rises in the abdomen, changes to globular shape |
| Umbilical cord, uterine bleeding | Cord protrudes and lengthens, blood may trickle or gush from behind, separating placenta with a loss of 250-300 mls |

| STAGES OF LABOR AND ASSOCIATED CHANGES ||
|---|---|
| Mechanism of placental expulsion | Separation from inner to outer margins (Duncan mechanism) or separation from outer margins, inward (Schultz Mechanism) |
| Cardiac output | Increases in response to UCs and changes in peripheral volume; increases 30% during labor, decreases 15%-25% after birth; BP and P return to normal during recovery hour |
| **Stage IV (Immediate postpartum)** | **Changes 1-2 hours after delivery** |
| Uterine height, tone position | Uterine fundus at umbilicus, positioned in midline; firm, contracted, or becomes firm when massaged |
| Lochia | Moderate amount of rubra; vaginal bleeding with occasional clots |
| Perineum | Episiotomy or laceration present; some soreness, edema, ecchymosis possible |

| STAGES OF LABOR AND ASSOCIATED CHANGES | |
|---|---|
| Bladder distention | Fullness may displace fundus upward and cause boggy or relaxed uterus |
| Breasts | Soft with erect nipples, breast feeding may start at this time |
| Vital signs | Some change in BP from anesthesia (lower) or medications (higher), pulse may be slower, temperature may be slightly elevated for 24 hours |

## BREATHING TECHNIQUES

Breathing techniques are used for relaxation in the early phases of labor. In second stage, breathing for pushing increases intra-abdominal pressure and aids in the delivery of the fetus.

**Dilatation to 3 cm**:
- Take cleansing breath (breathe in through the nose and out through the mouth with lips pursed.)
- Keep breathing slow and rhythmic, about 8-10 breaths per minute during each contraction.
- When the contraction ends, take one deep breath and then breathe normally.

**Dilatation 4-7 cm**:

- Take cleansing breath at the beginning of each contraction.

- Breathing becomes more shallow with a rate of about 16 per minute. (Caution against hyperventilation.)

- Encourage slow, abdominal breathing, especially in between contractions.

**Dilatation of 8-10 cm**:

- Always start with a cleansing breath.

- Maintain concentration or breathing as contractions intensify.

- Encourage use of 4:1 breathing pattern: breath, breath, breath, and puff.

- Panting breaths are encouraged to keep mother from pushing down before full dilation is achieved.

# FETAL MONITORING

| Stage | FHT range/method | FHT changes/ cause | Interventions |
|---|---|---|---|
| *Antepartum* | 120-160 bpm heard at 12 weeks with doppler, at 20 weeks with fetoscope | | Monitored at prenatal visits |
| *Intrapartum*<br><br>**Stage I Labor Latent Phase** | 120-160 bpm with fetoscope, electronic fetal monitoring (EFM) | Variability in rate during fetal movement and uterine contractions. Baseline of 120 bpm to 160 bpm (Bradycardia is a baseline less than 120 bpm and Tachycardia is a baseline greater than 160 bpm) | Usually heard below umbilicus taken by fetoscope to identify baseline. Requires continuous electronic fetal monitoring and action for late deceleration |

| Stage 1 Labor Active Transition Phases | 120-160 bpm with fetoscope, EFM | Some rate variations in response to fetal movement and contractions; decelerations or accelerations detected with electronic fetal monitoring | Heard below umbilicus based on fetal descent |
|---|---|---|---|
| Early Deceleration | Rate usually in normal range (120-160 bpm) | Early deceleration caused by fetal head compression descent with 1 cm/hr primigravida; 2 cm/hr multipara | Assess tracing for onset early in contraction, return to baseline by end of contraction. Compare tracing with FHT by doptone, contractions by palpation |

| | | | |
|---|---|---|---|
| **Late Deceleration** | Rate based on fetal hypoxia; usually in normal range of 120-130 bpm | Late deceleration caused by impaired uterine circulation | Assess tracing for slowing 20-30 seconds after start of contraction and return to baseline after end of contraction |
| **Variable Deceleration** | Rate based on cord compression; usually lower than normal range | Variable deceleration with abrupt onset; duration caused by degree or severity of cord compression | Assess for severity; change maternal position |
| **Repeated Late Decelerations** | Late decel: FHR in normal range; nonreassuring baseline variability; EFM | Late deceleration caused by placental insufficiency | $O_2$ with face mask @ 8 L/min; notify physician, prepare for immediate delivery if no improvement |

| | | | |
|---|---|---|---|
| **Severe Variable Decelerations** | Variable decel: FHR < 60 bpm or ≥ 60 bpm below baseline for ≥ 60 seconds; slow return to baseline | Variable decel caused by cord compression; both indicate fetal hypoxia | |
| **Stage II Labor Expulsion of fetus** | 120-160 bpm by fetoscope, continuous EFM | May vary 6-10 bpm during birth with bradycardia during contractions, with return to baseline after contraction; rate after birth 100 bpm unless infant is compromised by uterine/ placental insufficiency | Perform APGAR scoring 1 and 5 minutes after birth |

## DANGER SIGNS DURING LABOR

The labor and delivery nurse should be alert for any deviation from normal. The most common danger signs are:

* Intrauterine pressure above 75 mmHg

* Contractions occuring more than every 2 minutes before transition phase

* Contractions lasting longer than 60 seconds

* Fetal bradycardia or tachycardia

* Irregular fetal heart rate

* Absence of fetal heartbeat

* Bloody or greenish amniotic fluid

* Prolapsed umbilical cord

* Stop in the descent of the fetus

* Lack of progress in dilatation and/or effacement

## Apgar Scoring System

|  | 0 | 1 | 2 |
|---|---|---|---|
| **Heart Rate** | Absent | Slow (less than 100 beats/min.) | Greater than 100 beats/min. |
| **Respiratory Effort** | Absent | Slow or irregular | Good: crying lustily |
| **Muscle Tone** | Limp | Some flexion of extremities | Active motion: well flexed |
| **Reflex Irritability** | No response | Grimace | (Cough or sneeze); vigorous cry |
| **Color** | Blue or pale | Body pink, extremities blue | Completely pink |

## UMBILICAL CORD CARE

* Wipe stump area with alcohol soaked cotton ball every day to promote drying.

* Let area air dry.

* Fold diaper down to prevent contact with stump area.

* Observe for signs and symptoms of infection.

* Do not give tub bath until stump falls off.

* Stump usually falls off in 10 days.

* Do not, under any circumstances, attempt to forcefully remove the cord.

## CARDIOPULMONARY RESUSCITATION
## ONE RESCUER CPR, ADULT

| ASSESSMENT | ACTION |
|---|---|
| 1. **Airway**. Determine unresponsiveness. Call for help. Position victim. Open airway. | Shake shoulder, *"Are you ok?"* *Call out*, **"Help!"** Turn to supine position. Use head-tilt/chin-lift maneuver. |
| 2. **Breathing**. Determine breathlessness. Ventilate. | Ear over mouth, observe chest: look, listen. Feel for breathing *(35 seconds)*. Seal mouth and nose. Ventilate 2 times at a rate of 1-1.5 seconds per inspiration. Watch chest rise for adequate ventilation. |

3. **Circulation**. Determine pulselessness. Activate EMS. Begin chest compressions.

Check carotid 5-10 seconds. Maintain head-tilt. If someone has responded, send him or her for help or to call 911. Check landmark for hand placement two fingers above xyphoid process. Compress 1 1/2-2". Compression rate: 80-100 min.

4. **Compression**. Ventilation ratio.

15-2. 15 compressions and 2 ventilations. Do 4 cycles and check carotid (5 seconds). If no pulse, continue CPR.

## TWO RESCUER CPR,  ADULT

### ASSESSMENT                    ACTION

1. **Airway**.
*(Same procedure as one man.)*

2. **Breathing**.
*(Same procedure as one man.)*

3. **Circulation**. Determine pulselessness. Compressor gets into position.

Say "No pulse." Check landmark.

4. **Compression/ Ventilation ratio.**

Ratio: 5-1. Rate: 80-100/min. Say any mnemonic. Stop compression to allow for each ventilation. Ventilator ventilates after every 5 compressions. After 10 cycles, ventilator checks carotid pulse.

5. **Call for switch.**

Compressor calls for switch. Compressor completes 5th compression. Ventilator completes ventilation, then switches.

6. **Switch.**

Ventilator moves to chest and compressor moves to head in simultaneous movement. New ventilator checks carotid. Say, "No pulse," ventilate once. Continue CPR.

## ONE RESCUER CPR, INFANT

### ASSESSMENT

### ACTION

1. **Airway.**
*(Same procedure as one man adult.)*

Be careful not to hyperextend the head. Ventilate twice.

2. **Breathing** .
*(Same procedure as one man adult.)*

**EXCEPTION**: Make tight seal around nose and mouth. Do not force air (gently puff volume of air in your cheeks).

3. **Circulation.** Determine pulselessness. Activate EMS. Begin chest compression.

Feel for brachial pulse for 5-10 seconds. Draw imaginary line between nipples. Place 2 fingers on sternum, 1 finger's width below imaginary line. Compress vertically, 1/2-1". Say any helpful mnemonic. Compression rate: 100/min.

4. **Compression/ Ventilation ratio.**

Ratio: 5-1; 5 compressions to 1 slow ventilation. Pause for ventilation. Do ten cycles, then check brachial pulse. No pulse: ventilate once. Continue CPR.

## NEONATAL PHYSICAL ASSESSMENT

The physical assessment of the neonate is head-to-toe and involves the following components and anticipated findings:

| COMPONENT | ANTICIPATED FINDINGS |
|---|---|
| **Posture (at rest)** | Flexed extremities, clenched fists |
| **Body/Muscle tone** | Resists extension of extremities (assessed throughout) |
| **Moro Reflex** | Response to loud sound, loss of support |

| **COMPONENT** | **ANTICIPATED FINDINGS** |
|---|---|
| **Vital Signs** | |
| Temperature | 97-99° axillary |
| Heart rate | 120-160 bpm (at rest) |
| | 160-180 bpm (crying) |
| | 80-120 bpm (deep rest) |
| Respiratory rate | 30-60 rpm |
| | >60 rpm (crying) |
| **Vital statistics** | |
| Weight | 2500-4000 grams |
| | (5 lb 8 oz - 8 lb 13 oz) |
| | <2500 grams (SGA or preterm) |
| | >4000 grams (LGA) |
| Length | 18-22 inches (45-55 cm) |
| Head circumference | 12.5-13.75 inches (32-35 cm) |
| Chest circumference | 2 cm less than head circumference |
| Abdominal circumference | Approximately the same as chest |
| **Skin** | |
| Color | Pink or consistent with ethnicity |
| Lanugo | Amount (decreases with gestational age) |
| Turgor | Elastic |

| COMPONENT | ANTICIPATED FINDINGS |
|---|---|
| **Head** | |
| Molding | Overlapping suture lines present |
| Anterior fontanelle | Diamond shape (3-4 cm x 2-3 cm) |
| | Depressed in dehydration |
| | Bulging in intracranial pressure |
| Posterior fontanelle | Triangle shape (0.5-1.0 cm) |
| Hair | Fine, color |
| Face | Symmetry of features and movement |
| | Eyebrows and eyelashes present |
| Eyes | Blue, slate gray |
| | White sclera |
| | PERRLA, red reflex, blink reflex |
| Mouth | Epstein's pearls |
| | Intact hard and soft palate |
| | Uvula midline: root, suck, swallow, gag, extrusion reflexes |
| Nose | Nares patent (obligatory nose breather) |
| Milia | Present on face (bridge of nose, chin) |
| Ears | Symmetric |
| | Top in line with eye canthi |
| | Hearing (responds to sounds) |
| Head lag | 45° or less |

| COMPONENT | ANTICIPATED FINDINGS |
|---|---|
| **Neck** | |
| Mobility | Full range of motion |
| Thyroid gland | Nonpalpable |
| Lymph nodes | Nonpalpable |
| Clavicles | Intact |
| Control | Raises head when supine Brief control in erect position |
| Reflex | Tonic neck |
| **Chest** | |
| Shape | Cylindric, symmetric |
| Expansion | Symmetric, synchronous with abdomen |
| Auscultation | Lung sounds CTA (clear to auscultation) Heart sounds, rate, regular |
| PMI | Palpable & observable at 3rd-4th interspace |
| Breast | Palpable bud (5-10 mm) |
| Brachial pulses | Palpable, equal bilaterally Equal with PMI |
| **Abdomen** | |
| Shape | Round, symmetric |
| Umbilicus | 2 arteries, 1 vein No protrusion |
| Auscultation | Bowel sounds present @ 1-2 hours of life |

| COMPONENT | ANTICIPATED FINDINGS |
|---|---|
| Palpation | Slight diastasis recti |
| | Liver edge (@-1 cm below costal margin) |
| | Spleen (@-1 cm below left costal margin) |
| | Kidneys |
| Percussion | Liver, spleen size |
| Femoral pulse | Palpable equal bilaterally |
| | Equal with PMI |
| **Genitalia** | |
| Urination | First voiding within 24 hours of age |
| Labia | Majora > or cover minora |
| Vagina | Vaginal tag |
| | Mucous and/or bloody discharge |
| Penis | Meatus at tip |
| | Foreskin adherent to glans |
| Scrotum | Rugae, testes descended |
| **Back and Anus** | |
| Buttocks | Symmetrical |
| Spine | Straight, flexible |
| Alignment | Shoulders, scapulae, & iliac crests |
| Sacrum | Intact |
| Reflexes | Trunk incurvation, crossed extension |
| | Landau |

| COMPONENT | ANTICIPATED FINDINGS |
|---|---|
| Anus | Patent |
| | Meconium, transitional stools |
| | Wink reflex |
| **Extremities** | |
| Arms | Symmetry of movement |
| | Flexed at rest |
| | Equal length |
| | Moro reflex response |
| | Palmar grasp |
| Hands | Fingers separate, 5 each hand |
| | Finger nails present |
| | Palmar crease normal |
| Legs | Symmetry of movement |
| | Flexed at rest |
| | Equal length, symmetric skin folds |
| | Ortolani maneuver (no dislocation or clicks) |
| | Stepping reflex |
| Feet | Plantar sole creases |
| | 5 separate toes each foot |
| | Plantar grasp |
| | Babinski reflex |

# ASSESSMENT OF GESTATIONAL AGE

| Assessment Component | Value | Criteria |
|---|---|---|
| **Posture at rest** | 0 | Extension of all extremities |
| | 1 | Extension of arms |
| | | Beginning flexion of thighs |
| | 2 | Extension of arms |
| | | Beginning flexion of legs |
| | 3 | Beginning flexion of arms, flexion of legs |
| | 4 | Complete flexion of arms and legs |
| **Square Window** | -1 | >90° angle |
| | 0 | 90° angle (Hypothenar eminence & forearm) |
| | 1 | 60° angle |
| | 2 | 45° angle |
| | 3 | 30° angle |
| | 4 | 0° angle |
| **Arm recoil** | 0 | Arms remain extended |
| | 1 | 140°-180° angle (at elbow) |

| Assessment Component | Value | Criteria |
|---|---|---|
| Arm recoil (continued) | 2 | 110°-140° angle (at elbow) |
| | 3 | 90°-100° angle |
| | 4 | <90° angle |
| Popliteal angle | -1 | 180° angle (extension) |
| | 0 | 160° angle (behind the knee) |
| | 1 | 140° angle |
| | 2 | 120° angle |
| | 3 | 100° angle |
| | 4 | 90° angle |
| | 5 | <90° angle |
| Scarf sign | -1 | Elbow at opposite arm |
| | 0 | Elbow at opposite shoulder |
| | 1 | Elbow at opposite nipple |
| | 2 | Elbow at midline |
| | 3 | Elbow at same side nipple |
| | 4 | Elbow at same side shoulder |
| Heel to ear | -1 | Toes touch ear, 180° angle (behind knee) |

| Assessment Component | Value | Criteria |
|---|---|---|
| Heel to ear (continued) | 0 | Toes almost touch face |
| | 1 | 130° angle |
| | 2 | 110° angle |
| | 3 | 90° angle |
| | 4 | <90° angle |
| Physical maturity; skin | -1 | Sticky, friable, transparent skin |
| | 0 | Edematous extremities; gelatinous, red translucent skin |
| | 1 | Tibial edema |
| | | Smooth pink color |
| | | Visible veins |
| | 2 | No edema |
| | | Superficial peeling and/or rash |
| | | Few veins |
| | 3 | Cracking |
| | | Pale areas |
| | | Rare veins |
| | 4 | Deep cracking |
| | | Parchment-like skin |
| | | No vessels |
| | 5 | Cracked, wrinkled leathery |

| Assessment Component | Value | Criteria |
|---|---|---|
| **Lanugo** | -1 | None |
| | 0 | Sparse |
| | 1 | Abundant |
| | 2 | Thinning |
| | 3 | Bald areas |
| | 4 | Mostly bald |
| **Plantar crease** | -1 | Heel-to-toe 40-50 mm |
| | 0 | None |
| | 1 | Faint red marks (upper $1/2$ sole) |
| | 2 | Anterior transverse crease only |
| | 3 | Creases over anterior $2/3$ of sole |
| | 4 | Creases cover entire sole |
| **Breast** | -1 | Imperceptible |
| | 0 | Nipple barely perceptible |
| | | No palpable breast bud |
| | 1 | Nipple present |
| | | Flat areola |
| | | No palpable breast bud |

| Assessment Component | Value | Criteria |
|---|---|---|
| Breast (*continued*) | 2 | Stippled areola with flat edge |
| | | 1-2 mm breast bud |
| | 3 | Stippled areola with raised edge |
| | | 3-4 mm breast bud |
| | 4 | Full areola & 5-10 mm breast bud |
| Eye/Ear | -1 | Lids fused loosely |
| | 0 | Lids open, pinna flat (no cartilage); soft remains folded |
| | 1 | Slightly curved pinna, soft slow re-coil (unfolding) |
| | 2 | Well curved pinna, soft but ready recoil |
| | 3 | Formed pinna, firm to edge |
| | | Instant recoil |
| | 4 | Thick cartilage, ear stiff |
| Genitals: | | |
| Male | -1 | Scrotum flat, smooth |
| | 0 | No testes in scrotum, faint rugae present |

| Assessment Component | Value | Criteria |
|---|---|---|
| **Male** (*continued*) | 1 | Testes in upper canal; rare rugae |
| | 2 | Testes descending, few rugae |
| | 3 | Testes within scrotum, good rugae |
| | 4 | Testes in pendulous scrotum, rugae cover scrotum |
| **Female** | -1 | Clitoris prominent, labia flat |
| | 0 | Prominent clitoris and small labia minora |
| | 1 | Prominent clitoris, enlarging labia minora |
| | 2 | Labia majora & minora equally prominent |
| | 3 | Labia majora appear large, labia minora appear small |
| | 4 | Labia majora completely cover labia minora |

**TOTAL SCORE:** _____

## MATURITY RATING

Determined by comparing the total score with the corresponding weeks gestation according to the following values

| TOTAL SCORE | WEEKS GESTATION |
|---|---|
| -10 | 20 |
| -5 | 22 |
| 0 | 24 |
| 5 | 26 |
| 10 | 28 |
| 15 | 30 |
| 20 | 32 |
| 25 | 34 |
| 30 | 36 |
| 35 | 38 |
| 40 | 40 |
| 45 | 42 |
| 50 | 44 |

## ISOLATION PROCEDURES

Isolation techniques prevent dissemination of harmful pathogens to susceptible patients and/or health care workers by establishing barriers to these pathogens. The Center for Disease Control issues recommendations for isolation procedures; however, hospitals will establish their own protocols for following these recommendations Therefore, nurses may see wide variances in how the guidelines are implemented.

## ASSESSMENT

* Physician's orders and agency policy
* Medical diagnosis
* Isolation required

## EQUIPMENT

* Private room with door closed at all times
* Door sign with isolation level
* Linen gown
* Disposable gowns, masks, gloves, caps, goggles, and shoe covers
* Separate laundry hamper
* Waste container with plastic lining
* Antimicrobial soap
* Disposable, sterile utensils, dishes, tray
* Sterile linen, diagnostic tools, or any articles that will contact patient
* Isolation labels
* Preparation
* Wash hands and examine for breaks in skin
* Identify patient
* Assemble equipment
* Explain precautions and procedures to patient, family, and visitors
* Place isolation sign and instructions on door

## PROCEDURES

* For infected patient: gown, gloves, and mask according to isolation level. Elevate bed to working level. Carry out intended procedure or care of patient

* Provide appropriate containers for disposal of materials. Avoid vigorous movement of bed linen

* Dispose of all waste items including gloves, mask and paper gowns before leaving room

## RATIONALE

* Protects nurse from contamination

* Receives isolation materials

* Prevents dissemination of pathogens by area movement

* Contaminated items may not leave room until properly disposed

## PROCEDURES

With second nurse standing outside of room holding clean cuffed plastic bag, first nurse securely fastens plastic lined bag containing contaminated material. Red labels identify contents. Nurse outside room holds second bag open and first bag is dropped inside second bag

* Remove gowns before leaving room

* Wash hands before untying gown ties

* Remove gown inside out and roll up

* Before entering room, using strict medical asepsis, wash hands

## RATIONALE

∗ "Double bagging" decreases possibility of contamination to environment outside of patient's room

∗ Prevents transportation of pathogens

∗ Prevents spread of microorganisms

∗ Area of gown touching uniform is considered clean; by rolling, harmful pathogens are trapped inside

# ISOLATION LEVELS

*Strict*

Private room, gown, masks, gloves when entering, all articles in room considered contaminated. Use disposable dishes. Prevents dissemination by contact and airborne sources. Recommended most commonly in childhood diseases. Rarely used except for varicella (chickenpox), Zoster (shingles), smallpox, and diphtheria.

*Respiratory*

Private room, mask when in close contact with patient. Double bag linens and trash. All articles in room considered contaminated. Prevents dissemination by contact and airborne sources. Infections requiring respiratory isolation include measles, epiglottitis, meningitis, pneumonia, mumps, whooping cough (pertussis).

*Enteric*

Private room, gown and gloves if handling articles with feces and vomitus. Infection may spread by direct or indirect contact. Prevents dissemination by contact with contaminated articles or feces. Common infections requiring enteric isolation are amebic dysentery, cholera, diarrhea of unknown cause, encephalitis, Hepatitis A, viral meningitis and gastroenteritis.

## Blood/Body Fluid

Private room, gown and gloves if handling articles contaminated with blood or body fluids. Prevents dissemination by direct or indirect contact with blood or body fluids. Double bag linens and trash. Common infections requiring this isolation are AIDS, Hepatitis B and C, malaria and syphilis.

## Body Substance

Instituted in 1987, this procedure requires masks, gloves, gowns and goggles. It is a protection against any body substance, including sweat and tears. It has largely replaced respiratory isolation.

## AFB (Acid Fast Bacilli)

This is a new, highly-specialized isolation that recommends special ventilation of rooms and protective clothing. It focuses on preventing the spread of tuberculosis. Wear gown and masks if in direct contact: gloves are not necessary. Double bag linens and trash.

## Drainage/Secretion

Gown, gloves when handling drainage or secretion from any source. Prevents dissemination by contaminated articles. This procedure is not widely used because it has been incorporated into the blood/body fluid guidelines. Infections include draining wound infections such as abscesses, minor burns, decubitus ulcers and conjunctivas.

## Contact

Private room, gown, mask, gloves for anyone in contact with patient. All articles in contact with patient are considered contaminated. Prevents dissemination by contact and airborne sources. This is the next most strict isolation. Rarely used except in methicillin resistant infections. Infections requiring this isolation are diphtheria, some cases of influenza, impetigo, pediculosis (lice), staph or strep pneumonia, rabies, rubella, and scabies.

*Note: Protective or reverse isolation is not an official CDC category. However, physicians may order it on an individualized basis, especially for oncology patients. All levels require labeling and bagging of contaminated materials.*

# TEACHING TOPICS

# TEACHING TOPICS

Problems of Pregnancy and Interventions ................. 105

Signs of Labor ............................................................. 112

Pain Management During Labor ............................... 114

The Basic Four Food Pyramid Guide ....................... 116

Recommended Daily Allowances ............................... 119

Recommended Dietary Allowances ........................... 120

Recommended Nutrient Supplementation ................. 129

Food Sources of Nutrients ........................................ 131

Complications of Pregnancy and Treatments ........... 134

Hyperemesis Gravidarum .......................................... 136

Pregnancy-Induced Hypertension ............................. 137

Symptoms of PIH ...................................................... 138

Ectopic Pregnancy ..................................................... 140

The Puerperium .......................................................... 141

Maternal Comfort Measures ..................................... 143

Maternal Self-Care Measures ................................... 147

Infant Care Measures ................................................ 149

Guidelines for Calling Health Care Provider ........... 150

Adjustment to Parenting Role ................................... 151

Summary of Methods of Contraception .................... 152

# PROBLEMS OF PREGNANCY AND INTERVENTIONS

**First trimester**

*Problem*: Nausea, vomiting ("morning sickness")

*Interventions*:

Dry crackers, toast in AM; frequent, small meals; avoid offensive odors; eliminate highly-seasoned fried food; liquids with meals.

*Problem*: Malnutrition (obesity/underweight)

*Interventions*:

Provide a copy of the Food Pyramid and/or dietary lists of food inclusions to ensure adequate nutrition in pregnancy and weight gain of 25-35 pounds; provide reduction calories in overweight patients while maintaining nutrients; monitor weight gain.

*Problem*: Breast changes (soreness/enlargement)

*Interventions*:

Wear supportive bra night and day; expose nipples to air qd for 1/2 hour; avoid trauma, strong soaps.

*Problem*: Leukorrhea, excessive perspiration

*Interventions*:

Daily shower with mild soap, use deodorant and wear cotton undergarments.

***Problem***: Urinary frequency

***Interventions***.

Maintain close proximity to bathroom.


***Problem***:  Leg cramps, varicose veins

***Interventions***.

Stretch leg muscles; exercise by walking; elevate/extend legs when sitting; position foot in dorsiflexion; avoid standing in one place for long periods of time, crossing legs, wearing garters.


***Problem***: Vertigo, headaches

***Interventions***.

Monitor BP for elevation, position on left side when lying down, change position slowly.


***Problem***:  Fatigue

***Interventions***.

Rest periods during day; use of relaxation techniques.


***Problem***: Nasal stuffiness, epistaxis

***Interventions***.

Avoid blowing nose hard; provide humidification; avoid nasal/decongestion sprays; lower head; apply ice to back of neck or apply pressure to nose if bleeding occurs.

*Problem*:  Dyspareunia

*Interventions*:

Teach that decreased interest in sexual activity and responsiveness are normal; suggest position changes that might decrease discomfort.


*Problem*:  Use of drugs, alcohol, smoking

*Interventions*:

Teach hazards of these practices or conditions; risk of sexually transmitted diseases to the fetus; refer to counseling, treatment, rehabilitation.


**Second trimester**:

*Problem*:  Chloasma ("mask of pregnancy"),  striae gravidarum, body shape changes

*Interventions*:

Teach that these changes are normal, suggest clothing and makeup that will enhance appearance.


*Problem*:  Backache

*Interventions*:

Teach pelvic tilt exercises, suggest wearing low-heeled shoes, avoid belts/restrictive clothing.

*Problem*: Inadequate exercise

*Interventions*:

Teach body mechanics and correct posture, importance of walking; suggest sit-ups, squatting, stretch/press exercises, walking posture; Kegel's exercises.

**Third trimester:**

*Problem*: Edema (dependent/generalized)

*Interventions*:

Avoid constrictive clothing, sitting or standing for long periods of time; elevate feet when sitting, assume side-lying position for sleep, avoid adding salt to foods; maintain comfortable room temperature.

*Problem*: Difficulty breathing

*Interventions*:

Use pillows to elevate head and chest for sleep, avoid eating large meals, teach good posture, breathing changes are normal.

*Problem*: Pyrosis, bloating, flatulence

*Interventions*:

Avoid gas-forming, greasy/fried foods, hot/cold foods; teach to eat small meals more frequently; maintain upright position during and after eating; chew gum; suck hard candy; suggest antacid if approved by physician.

**Problem:** Constipation, hemorrhoids

**Interventions:**

Dietary inclusion of fiber; fluid intake 8-10 glasses/day; walking/exercises within limits; stool softener as prescribed; avoid laxatives/enemas; provide sitz baths; topical anesthesia ointment to anal area; using gloved finger, reinsert hemorrhoids as needed.

**Problem:** Sleep disturbance, insomnia

**Interventions:**

Suggest naps during the day, positions for sleep using pillows for support, warm shower, reading, relaxation exercises before H.S.

**Problem:** Urinary frequency

**Interventions:**

Reduce fluid intake before H.S., avoid prolonged upright/supine positions, maintain proximity to bathroom.

**Problem:** Anxiety about labor, welfare of infant

**Interventions:**

Teach stages of labor, contraction characteristics and timing, differences between Braxton-Hicks contractions and those indicating labor. Teach relaxation and coping techniques. Suggest childbirth education classes

### Postpartum

***Problem:***  Involution

***Interventions:***

Teach that uterine fundus decreases in size qd after initial 24 hour period until normal size occurs in 4-6 weeks; massage fundus to maintain tone, maintain urinary elimination to prevent bladder distention.

***Problem:***  Pain ("after pains")

***Interventions:***

Mild analgesic as prescribed, teach that pain occurs more intensely in multipara and increases in severity with increased number of births. It also occurs with breastfeeding. The discomfort occurs for the first 2-3 days postpartum.

***Problem:***  Lochia

***Interventions:***

Teach that rubra (red) is present for 2-3 days, serous (brownish) 3-10 days, then alba (yellowish-white); report excessive or foul-smelling lochia.

***Problem:***  Urinary retention

***Interventions:***

Monitor I&O, suggest voiding q3h, allow water to run, pour warm water over genitalia, encourage to void during shower if urge present, fluid intake of 6-8 glasses/day, catheterize only if needed, perform Kegel's exercises.

*Problem:*  Episiotomy, hemorrhoids

*Interventions:*

Apply ice pack, cleanse from front to back after elimination, change pad after each elimination; provide
moist heat (sitz bath) after 12-24 hours, 2-4 times per
day, local anesthesia ointment, spray; compresses to
area; teach positions for sitting to avoid discomfort.

*Problem:*  Breast engorgement

*Interventions:*

If bottle feeding, apply ice pack, wear supportive bra
or binder, avoid actions that stimulate nipples.  Teach
breast and nipple care if nursing (cleansing, air exposure, use of nursing pads, application of ointment, use
of breast pump and early initiation of breastfeeding).

*Problem:*  Postpartum depression

*Interventions:*

Allow expression of feelings, teach and support abilities
to care for infant, teach that feeling depressed is normal after birth, provide privacy for nonverbal expression of feelings (crying, irritability, mood changes)
involve in planning care for infant, monitor for signs of
postpartum psychosis, refer to counseling if needed.

*Problem:*  Weight loss

*Interventions:*

Inform of usual weight loss after birth (about 17
pounds); provide weight reduction diet if overweight,

taking into consideration lactation and postpartum recovery needs.

# SIGNS OF LABOR

Premonitory signs of labor occur several hours to several days before the onset of labor and act as an advanced warning or "premonition" that labor is impending. The signs include:

**Lightening**: The beginning of descent of the fetus into the pelvis. It occurs in primigravid mothers 2-3 weeks before the onset of labor and may not occur in multiparous mothers until sometime in the labor process.

**Braxton-Hicks contractions**: The irregular, intermittent, mild uterine contractions that have been occurring throughout pregnancy but were undetected by the expectant mother until near term. They become increasingly stronger until they cause maternal discomfort. Although they are frequently confused as the beginning of labor, they do not produce progressive change in the cervix, and they are, therefore, termed "false labor contractions."

**Cervical changes**: The cervix becomes softer; initial effacement, and initial dilation begin to occur a few days before the onset of labor.

**Bloody show**: Bloody show, which is noticed with passage of the mucous plug, consists of a small amount of blood mixed with mucous, and is pinkish in color.

This sign usually occurs a few hours before the onset of labor.

**Burst of energy**: A few hours or days before the onset of labor. The mother suddenly feels very energetic and may be motivated to complete house cleaning, baking, and other activities previously omitted because of feelings of fatigue. The energy should be saved for labor.

**Spontaneous rupture of membranes**: A sudden gush of fluid escaping from the vagina which cannot be controlled by the mother. It can occur 12-24 hours before the onset of labor, or it may not occur until labor is well-established

## False Labor Signs

False labor signs are characteristics of uterine contractions that the expectant mother notices. However, the false labor contractions do not cause a progressive change in the cervix. The characteristics include the following:

- Contractions are irregular
- Pain is focused in the abdomen
- No significant change in duration, frequency, or intensity
- No change in cervical dilatation or effacement
- No change in intensity with walking

## True Labor Signs

The true labor signs are characteristics of uterine contractions noticed by the expectant mother and when assessed by a health care provider are determined to cause progressive change (effacement and dilatation) in the cervix. The characteristics include the following:

- Contractions occur at regular intervals
- Duration of contractions lengthens
- Pain begins in back and radiates to abdomen
- Intensity strengthens
- Time between contractions progressively shortens
- Intensity of contractions increases with walking
- Dilatation and effacement steadily progress

# PAIN MANAGEMENT DURING LABOR

* Encourage relaxation and breathing techniques throughout labor.

* Encourage walking, especially during early labor.

* Allow mother to assume the position in which she feels more comfortable.

* Do not mention the word "pain." Speak in terms of progress, dilatation, and contractions.

* Use pillows for support when mother is lying down. She should not lie supine during labor because of the pressure this position puts on the major blood vessels.

* Offer backrub and encourage significant other to massage (especially effleurage and touch).

* Offer ice chips, cold washcloths.

* Help mother conserve energy; do not ask unnecessary questions and "make conversation."

* Encourage mother to urinate frequently. (A full bladder may slow descent of the fetus.)

* Keep mother informed of fetal position, station, fetal heartbeat, dilatation, and effacement.

* Encourage rest between contractions, even a nap if possible.

* Do not perform procedures during contractions.

* Provide emotional support to mother and significant other.

* Assess need for pain medication, especially during the transitional period.

# USDA FOOD GUIDE PYRAMID

## A Guide to Daily Food Choices

The Pyramid is an outline of what to eat each day. It's not a rigid prescription, but a general guide that lets you choose a healthful diet that's right for you. The Pyramid calls for eating a variety of foods to get the nutrients you need and at the same time the right amount of calories to maintain a healthy weight.

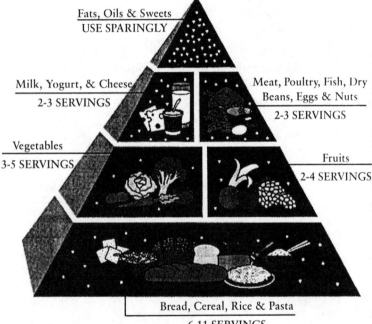

Fats, Oils & Sweets
USE SPARINGLY

Milk, Yogurt, & Cheese
2-3 SERVINGS

Meat, Poultry, Fish, Dry Beans, Eggs & Nuts
2-3 SERVINGS

Vegetables
3-5 SERVINGS

Fruits
2-4 SERVINGS

Bread, Cereal, Rice & Pasta
6-11 SERVINGS

The FOOD GUIDE PYRAMID emphasizes foods from the five food groups shown in three lower sections of the Pyramid.

Each of these food groups provides some, but not all, of the nutrients you need. Foods in one group can't replace those in another. No one food group is more important than another– for good health, you need them all.

Source: U.S. DEPARTMENT OF AGRICULTURE and the U.S. DEPARTMENT OF HEALTH AND HUMAN SERVICE
Provided by: the Education Department of the NATIONAL LIVE STOCK AND MEAT BOARD

| FOOD GROUP | SERVINGS DURING PREGNANCY | SERVINGS DURING LACTATION |
|---|---|---|
| **Dairy Products** | **Four 8-oz cups** | **Four 8-oz cups** |
| Milk<br>Cheese<br>Yogurt<br>Cottage cheese<br>Ice cream | 1 cup milk =<br>1 1/2 oz cheese<br>1 c. yogurt<br>1 1/2 c. cottage cheese<br>1 1/2 c. ice cream | |
| **Meat Group** | **Three servings** | **Two servings** |
| Beef<br>Pork<br>Poultry<br>Fish<br>Eggs<br>Legumes<br>Nuts<br>Seeds<br>Peanut butter | 1 serving = 2 oz<br>1 serving =<br>1/2 c. legumes<br>1 T. peanut butter<br>1 egg | |
| **Grain Products** | **Six to eleven servings** | **Six to eleven servings** |
| Breads<br>Cereal<br>Pasta<br>Rice | 1 serving =<br>1 slice bread<br>3/4 c. or 1 oz cereal<br>1/2 c. pasta<br>1/2 c. rice | |

| Fruits | Two to four servings | Two to four servings |
|---|---|---|
| Citrus fruits<br>Berries<br>Melons | 1 serving =<br>1 medium fruit,<br>$1/2$-1 cup fruit | |
| **Vegetables** | **Three to five servings** | **Three to five servings** |
| Leafy green vegetables; deep yellow vegetables:<br>    Carrots<br>    Sweet potatoes<br>    Squash<br>    Tomatoes<br>Green vegetables:<br>    Peas<br>    Green beans<br>    Broccoli<br>    Beets<br>    Cabbage<br>    Potatoes<br>    Corn | (At least one serving of dark green or deep yellow vegetable for vitamin A)<br>One serving = $1/2$ - 1 c. vegetable, 2 tomatoes, 1 medium potato | |
| **Fats*** | **One serving** | **One serving** |
| Butter<br>Cream<br>Nuts<br>Cream cheese<br>Avocadoes<br>Oil | One serving = 1 tsp butter<br>2 T. cream<br>1 oz. cream cheese<br>1 med. avocado | |

*Fats are essential because they supply Vitamins A and D and essential fatty acids, especially linoleic acid. Daily needs are satisfied by small amounts of fat.

## RECOMMENDED DAILY
## ALLOWANCES FOR WOMEN

|  | 15-18 Yr | 19-24 Yr | 25-50 Yr |
|---|---|---|---|
| Energy (kcal) | 2,200 | 2,200 | 2,200 |
| Protein (gm) | 44 | 46 | 50 |
| Vitamin A (µg RE) | 800 | 800 | 800 |
| Vitamin D (µg) | 10 | 10 | 10 |
| Vitamin E (mg α-TE) | 8 | 8 | 8 |
| Vitamin K (µg) | 55 | 60 | 65 |
| Vitamin C (mg) | 60 | 60 | 60 |
| Thiamin (mg) | 1.1 | 1.1 | 1.1 |
| Riboflavin (mg) | 1.3 | 1.3 | 1.3 |
| Niacin (mg NE) | 15 | 15 | 15 |
| Vitamin $B_6$ (mg) | 1.5 | 1.6 | 1.6 |
| Folate (µg) | 180 | 180 | 180 |
| Vitamin $B_{12}$ (µg) | 2 | 2 | 2 |
| Calcium (mg) | 1,200 | 1,200 | 800 |
| Phosphorous (mg) | 1,200 | 1,200 | 800 |
| Magnesium (mg) | 300 | 280 | 280 |
| Iron (mg) | 15 | 15 | 15 |
| Zinc (mg) | 12 | 12 | 12 |
| Iodine (µg) | 150 | 150 | 150 |
| Selenium (µg) | 50 | 50 | 50 |

## RECOMMENDED DIETARY ALLOWANCES FOR PREGNANT AND LACTATING WOMEN

| | Pregnant | LACTATING | |
|---|---|---|---|
| | | 1st 6 mos. | 2nd 6 mos. |
| Energy (kcal) | + 0 1st tri<br>+300 2nd tri<br>+300 3rd tri | +500 | +500 |
| Protein  (gm) | 60 | 65 | 62 |
| Vitamin A ($\mu$g RE) | 800 | 1,300 | 1,200 |
| Vitamin D ($\mu$g) | 10 | 10 | 10 |
| Vitamin E (mg $\alpha$-TE) | 10 | 12 | 11 |
| Vitamin K ($\mu$g) | 65 | 65 | 65 |
| Vitamin C  (mg) | 70 | 95 | 90 |
| Thiamin  (mg) | 1.5 | 1.6 | 1.6 |
| Riboflavin  (mg) | 1.6 | 1.8 | 1.7 |
| Niacin  (mg NE) | 17 | 20 | 20 |
| Vitamin $B_6$ (mg) | 2.2 | 2.1 | 2.1 |
| Folate ($\mu$g) | 400 | 280 | 260 |
| Vitamin $B_{12}$ ($\mu$g) | 2.2 | 2.6 | 2.6 |
| Calcium (mg) | 1,200 | 1,200 | 1,200 |
| Phosphorous (mg) | 1,200 | 1,200 | 1,200 |
| Magnesium  (mg) | 320 | 355 | 340 |
| Iron  (mg) | 30 | 15 | 15 |
| Zinc  (mg) | 15 | 19 | 16 |
| Iodine  ($\mu$g) | 175 | 200 | 200 |
| Selenium  ($\mu$g) | 65 | 75 | 75 |

| Nutrient | Food Sources | Major Function |
|----------|--------------|----------------|
| **Protein** | Complete protein from animal sources: <br> Cheese <br> Meat <br> Milk <br> Fish <br> Poultry <br> Eggs <br> Incomplete protein (from plant sources): <br> Peas <br> Beans <br> Rice <br> Bread <br> Cereal <br> Nuts <br> Complementary protein: <br> Eggs and toast <br> Cornbread and milk <br> Beans and rice <br> Spaghetti and meat sauce | Builds and maintains all body tissues; builds blood; aids in formation of antibodies; provides energy after carbohydrates and fat supplies are exhausted |

| Nutrient | Food Sources | Major Function |
|----------|--------------|----------------|
| **Carbohydrates (Complex)** | Breads Cereals Rice Pasta Potatoes Corn Fruits Vegetables | Body's major source of energy; helps body utilize other nutrients |
| **(Simple)** | Sugar Honey, cookies Cake, pie Candy | |
| **Iron (Absorption blocked by milk)** | Red meats Enriched cereal, especially Malt-o-Meal Oatmeal Apricots Clams Prunes Liver Beans Legumes Almonds Wheat germ Spinach | Required for RBC reproduction; heme in iron required for proper $O_2$-carrying RBCs; required in pregnancy related to marked increase in blood volume; prevents iron-deficiency anemia; fetal iron storage in the liver |

| Nutrient | Food Sources | Major Function |
|----------|--------------|----------------|
| **Vitamin A** | Beef liver<br>Sweet potatoes<br>Carrots<br>Spinach<br>Cantaloupe<br>Apricots<br>Broccoli<br>Asparagus<br>Cheese | Maintains healthy skin, hair, mucous membranes; repairs tissue, especially epithelial cells; aids in bone growth and teeth development; helps body resist infection; essential for RNA reproduction and synthesis |
| **Vitamin B$_1$ (Thiamin)** | Poultry<br>Pork<br>Liver<br>Milk<br>Legumes<br>Breads (enriched)<br>Cereals (enriched)<br>Eggs | Essential for maintenance of circulation, digestion and nervous system; maintains metabolic functions |
| **Vitamin B$_2$ (Riboflavin)** | Beef liver<br>Milk<br>Steak<br>Ricotta cheese<br>Cottage cheese<br>Spinach<br>Brewer's yeast<br>Broccoli<br>Salmon<br>Turkey | Essential for formation of RBC's and antibodies; assists in metabolic function; aids in building nerve structures; helps cells to utilize oxygen |

| Nutrient | Food Sources | Major Function |
|---|---|---|
| **Vitamin B$_6$ (Pyridoxine)** | Meat<br>Liver<br>Whole grains<br>Deep green vegetables | Maintains antibody function; essential for RNA and DNA synthesis; critical for hemoglobin production; helps maintain sodium and potassium balance; balances nervous system function; aids in tryptophan conversion |
| **Vitamin B$_{12}$ (Cobalamin)** | Beef<br>Eggs<br>Milk<br>Fish<br>Pork<br>Liver | Essential for blood cell formation; maintains healthy nervous system; aids in iron absorption; prevents megaloblastic anemia |

| Nutrient | Food Sources | Major Function |
|----------|--------------|----------------|
| **Vitamin C** | Tomatoes<br>Citrus fruits<br>Broccoli<br>Strawberries<br>Green peppers<br>Potatoes<br>Green leafy<br>vegetables | Essential for collagen production; assists in bone and teeth formation; essential for healing processes; essential in RBC formation; aids in resistance to infections |
| **Vitamin D** | Egg yolk<br>Liver<br>Milk (fortified)<br>Salmon<br>Tuna<br>Sunlight | Necessary for absorption of calcium; maintains healthy skin, hair, mucous membranes; essential for formation of bones; plays a role in blood clotting mechanisms |

| Nutrient | Food Sources | Major Function |
|----------|--------------|----------------|
| **Vitamin E** | Butter<br>Eggs<br>Fruit<br>Nuts<br>Oil<br>Wheat germ<br>Vegetables | Maintains integrity of muscles and nerves; acts as an antioxidant in protecting other nutrients, especially vitamins A and C; prevents hemolysis of RBCs |
| **Vitamin K** | Liver<br>Green, leafy vegetables | Essential for coagulation of blood |
| **Folic acid** | Broccoli<br>Asparagus<br>Artichokes<br>Green, leafy vegetables<br>Whole grains<br>Legumes<br>Orange juice<br>Wheat germ | Maintains cell growth and reproduction; essential for RBC formation; essential for DNA production; aids in protein metabolism; prevents megaloblastic anemia |

| Nutrient | Food Sources | Major Function |
|---|---|---|
| **Niacin** | Meat<br>Eggs<br>Lean meat<br>Liver<br>Poultry<br>Seafood<br>Whole grains<br>Peanuts | Aids in circulation; aids in growth of body tissues; maintains metabolism; essential in sex hormone production |
| **Phosphorus** | Meat<br>Fish<br>Poultry<br>Nuts<br>Cheese<br>Whole grains<br>Phosphates in processed food | Maintains bones and teeth; regulates heart beat; assists in maintaining kidney function; pairs with calcium |
| **Sodium** | Table salt<br>Soy sauce<br>Seafood<br>Cured meats<br>Cheese<br>Processed foods | Maintains fluid balance; aids in functioning of nerves and muscles |
| **Potassium** | Meat<br>Bran<br>Potatoes<br>Broccoli<br>Bananas<br>Peanut butter<br>Green, leafy vegetables | Regulates heartbeat; works with sodium to maintain fluid balance; stimulates nerve impulses |

| Nutrient | Food Sources | Major Function |
|----------|--------------|----------------|
| **Zinc** | Shellfish<br>Meat<br>Liver<br>Eggs<br>Wheat bran | Maintains growth of sexual organs; essential for production of enzymes; aids in healing processes |
| **Fats** | Butter<br>Egg yolks<br>Fat in meat<br>Bacon<br>Milk<br>Eggs<br>Nuts | Supplies secondary source of energy; supplies essential fatty acids, especially linoleic acid |
| **Calcium** | Milk<br>Cheese<br>Salmon<br>Sardines<br>Nuts<br>Beans<br>Legumes<br>Dried fruits<br>Dark green, leafy vegetables | Essential for formation of bones and teeth; maintains blood clotting mechanisms; regulates heartbeat; plays a role in growth of muscle tissue |

## RECOMMENDATIONS FOR NUTRIENT
## SUPPLEMENTATION DURING PREGNANCY

| Supplement | Amount/Day | Indications |
|---|---|---|
| Iron* | 30 mg | All pregnant women during 2nd and 3rd trimesters |
| Folate* | 300 mcg | Pregnant women with inadequate intake of dietary folate |
| **Multivitamin/Mineral Preparation*** | | |
| Iron | 30 mg | Pregnant women with inadequate diets or in high-risk categories such as multiple pregnancy, heavy cigarette smoking, or alcohol/drug abuse |
| Zinc | 15 mg | |
| Copper | 2 mg | |
| Calcium | 250 mg | |
| Vitamin B6 | 2 mg | |
| Folate | 300 mcg | |
| Vitamin C | 50 mg | |
| Vitamin D | 5 mcg | |
| Vitamin D | 10 mcg (400 IU) | Complete vegetarians and women with low intake of Vitamin D-fortified milk |

| Supplement | Amount/Day | Indications |
|---|---|---|
| **Calcium\*\*** | 600 mg | Pregnant women under age 25 whose normal dietary intake is less than 600 mg/day |
| **Vitamin B$_{12}$** | 2 mcg | Complete vegetarians |
| **Zinc and Copper** | 15 mg 2 mg | Women taking therapeutic iron supplementation |

*Taken between meals or at bedtime on empty stomach*

*\*Taken at mealtime*

## APPROXIMATE CAFFEINE CONTENT OF 1 CUP (8OZ) OF BEVERAGE

| Beverage | Caffeine, mg |
|---|---|
| Coffee: Brewed | 75-150 |
| Coffee: Instant | 30-80 |
| Tea | 40-60 |
| Cola | 30-60 |
| Cocoa | 2-40 |

# FOOD SOURCES OF NUTRIENTS

## High-Sodium Foods

- Barbecue sauce
- Butter/margarine
- Canned seafood
- Cured meats
- Canned spaghetti sauce
- Buttermilk
- Canned chili
- Canned soups
- Dry onion soup mix
- Baking mixes (pancakes, muffins)

## Low-Sodium Foods

- Canned pumpkin
- Egg white and yolk
- Fruit
- Honey
- Lean meats
- Red kidney/lima beans
- Puffed wheat/rice
- Unsalted nuts
- Cooked turnips
- Fresh vegetables
- Grits (not instant)
- Jams and jellies
- Macaroons
- Baked/broiled poultry
- Sherbet
- Potatoes

## "Fast" Foods

- Macaroni and cheese
- Parmesan cheese
- Potato salad
- Sauerkraut
- TV dinners
- Microwave dinners
- Pickles
- Pretzels, potato chips
- Tomato ketchup

## Calcium-Rich Foods

- Bok choy
- Cheese
- Cream soups
- Canned salmon/sardines
- Molasses (blackstrap)
- Broccoli
- Almonds
- Kale
- Tofu
- Milk/ice cream

## Potassium-Rich Foods

- Avocados
- Broccoli
- Dried fruits
- Lima beans
- Navy beans
- Peaches
- Prunes
- Sunflower seeds
- Tomatoes
- Bananas
- Cantaloupe
- Grapefruit
- Nuts
- Oranges
- Potatoes
- Rhubarb
- Spinach

## Vitamin K-Rich Foods

- Asparagus
- Broccoli
- Cabbage
- Cheeses
- Fish
- Mustard greens
- Brussel sprouts
- Collards
- Milk
- Spinach
- Turnips
- Liver

## Iron-Rich Foods

- Cereals (enriched)
- Dried fruit
- Red meats (lean)
- Leafy green vegetables
- Legumes
- Eggs
- Shellfish
- Liver

## Foods that Acidify Urine

- Breads (whole grain)
- Cheeses
- Eggs
- Meats
- Poultry
- Cereals
- Cranberries
- Fish
- Plums
- Prunes

## Foods that Alkalinize Urine

- All fruits except cranberries, prunes, plums
- All vegetables
- Milk

## Foods Containing Tyramine

(Stimulate release of epinephrine and norepinephrine)

- Aged cheeses
- Bananas
- Bologna (aged meat)
- Chocolate
- Over-ripe fruit
- Smoked or pickled fish
- Avocados
- Yeasts
- Yogurt
- Liver
- Alcohol

# COMPLICATIONS OF PREGNANCY AND TREATMENTS

## PROBLEMS WITH THE PLACENTA

Abruptio placentae (premature separation of a normally implanted placenta) or placenta previa (abnormal implantation of the placenta in the lower uterine segment near or over the cervical os) are most often the cause of latter pregnancy hemorrhage. The following chart lists the symptoms of these two complications of pregnancy:

### Symptoms of Abruptio Placentae

* Absent to severe pain

* Concealed or obvious bleeding

* Dark red blood if obvious

* Bleeding continuous if obvious

* Uterine tone normal to boardlike

* Fetal position normal

* Fetal position abnormal

* Shock absent to severe

* PIH common

* Coagulopathy occasional to common

* History of abdominal trauma, hypertension, smoking, alcohol or cocaine use and previous abruptio placentae

* Increase in fundal height or change in uterine contour due to bleeding

## Nursing Interventions

* Infuse IV, prepare to administer blood
* Type and crossmatch
* Monitor FHR
* Insert Foley
* Measure degree of hemorrhage; count pads or weigh Chux (1g = 1 ml blood)
* Report signs/symptoms of DIC
* Monitor vital signs for shock
* Strict I&O
* Monitor CVP
* Provide supportive therapy in an emergency situation

## Symptoms of Placenta Previa

* No pain
* Small to heavy bleeding
* Bright red blood
* No increase in fundal due to bleeding
* Normal uterine tone
* Bleeding intermittent
* Shock (occasional)
* PIH not usual
* Coagulopathy rare

### Nursing Interventions

* Bedrest
* Prepare to induce labor if cervix is ripe (low-lying or partial placenta previa)
* Prepare for Cesarean birth (total placenta previa)
* Monitor vital signs and FHR
* Type and crossmatch in case blood is required
* Administer IV
* No vaginal (or rectal) exams
* Monitor blood loss

## HYPEREMESIS GRAVIDARUM

Hyperemesis gravidarum is excessive nausea and vomiting of pregnancy resulting in electrolyte, nutritional, and metabolic imbalances. Possibly caused by elevated estrogen levels and the higher HCG levels of the first trimester, especially increased with multiple gestation and hydatidiform mole, the disorder is often corrected with restoration of the imbalances and completion of the first trimester. With proper intervention, the outcome is essentially the same as for pregnancies without hyperemesis gravidarum. If the imbalances are not corrected, however, intrauterine growth retardation, CNS malformations, and embryonic/fetal death may be the outcome for the neonate.

### Symptoms of Hyperemesis Gravidarum

* Vomiting of all intake
* Retching between oral intake
* Dehydration
* Fluid and electrolyte imbalances

* Hypotension
* Tachycardia
* Increased hematocrit and BUN
* Oliguria
* Metabolic alkalosis followed by acidosis (prolonged vomiting)
* Weight loss
* Jaundice
* Starvation

### Nursing Interventions

* Administer IV fluids, at least 3000 ml/day, and parenteral vitamins
* Monitor strict I&O
* When oral intake is allowed, provide 6 small meals with plenty of liquids
* Administer Phenergan IM for nausea and vomiting
* NPO for first 48 hours
* Oral hygiene
* Quite, calm environment

## PREGNANCY-INDUCED HYPERTENSION

PIH (Pregnancy-Induced Hypertension), is a disorder characterized by hypertension, proteinuria, and edema. Based on severity of symptoms, PIH is classified as mild or severe preeclampsia, HELLP syndrome, or eclampsia (when convulsions occur). HELLP (Hemolysis, Elevated Liver enzymes, and Low Platelet count) Syndrome occurs in some cases of severe preeclampsia.

## Symptoms of PIH

**Mild preeclampsia:**

* Hypertension (increase of 30/15 mmHg or more above baseline or BP 140/90)
* Proteinuria (between 1+ and 2+ by dipstick)
* Edema (dependent plus puffiness of fingers and face)
* Reflexes (3+ but no clonus)
* Weight gain (>1 lb/week)

**Severe Preeclampsia:**

* Hypertension (160/110 mmHg or more)
* Proteinuria (2+ or greater by dip stick)
* Edema (generalized, pulmonary edema)
* Reflexes (3+ or greater with ankle clonus)
* Weight gain (>1 lb/week; may be sudden increase)
* Oliguria (< 30 ml/hour)
* Severe headache
* Visual disturbances (blurred, photophobia, spots)
* Severe irritability
* Epigastric pain
* Elevated serum creatinine
* Thrombocytopenia
* AST markedly elevated
* Increased hematocrit (hemoconcentration)

**Eclampsia:**
* Symptoms of severe preeclampsia
* Convulsions

**HELLP syndrome:**
* Symptoms of PIH
* AST and ALT elevated
* Platelet count (< 100,000/cubic mm))
* BUN and creatinine elevated
* Schistocytes or burr cells on peripheral smear
* Nausea and vomiting

### Nursing Interventions (Hospital Care)

* Diet high in protein (80 g/day to replace protein in urine)
* Bedrest
* Left lateral position (to decrease pressure on vena cava and increase general circulation)
* Administer magnesium sulfate (prevent convulsions)
* Be prepared to administer calcium gluconate as an antidote, if required
* Moderate sodium intake
* Monitor FHR, BP, serum magnesium levels, magnesium toxicity, breath sounds, DTRs
* Daily weight

* Monitor LOC to note impending convulsion
* Monitor fetal movement
* May administer diazepam (Valium) as a sedative
* Administer hydralazine (Apresoline) to lower diastolic blood pressure (for severe hypertension)
* Observe for vaginal bleeding
* Provide psychological support

## ECTOPIC PREGNANCY

Ectopic pregnancy occurs when gestation takes place outside the uterus—often in the ampullar or isthmus section of the fallopian tube. Ectopic pregnancy is a leading cause of death of pregnant women in the United States.

### Symptoms of Tubal Pregnancy

**Unruptured**:
* Missed period
* Adnexal fullness and tenderness
* Early symptoms of pregnancy
* Abdominal pain within 3-5 weeks of missed period (may be generalized or one-sided)
* Vague discomfort
* Scant, dark brown vaginal bleeding
* Positive serum pregnancy test

**Rupture:**

* Syncope

* Abdominal pain (may be sudden, sharp, severe)

* Shoulder pain (indicative of intraperitoneal bleeding that extends to diaphragm and phrenic nerve)

* Signs of hypovolemic shock

* Cullen's sign (blue tinge around umbilicus)

### Nursing Interventions

* Vital signs

* Administer IV fluids (especially for hypovolemia)

* Monitor vaginal bleeding

* Monitor signs/symptoms of hypovolemic shock

* RhoGAM (Rh negative client)

* Prepare laporoscopy or laparotomy

* Provide psychological support

## The Puerperium

## Developmental Changes of the Puerperium

The developmental changes of the puerperium involve the taking-in phase, the taking-hold phase and the letting-go phase. The characteristics of each are summarized below:

### Characteristics of the taking-in phase:

* Passivity
* Dependence on others
* Low energy level
* Hesitant in making decisions
* Relives labor and birth experience
* Preoccupied with self-needs
* Phase lasts one to three days in primigravida, perhaps only a few hours in multigravida

### Characteristics of the taking-hold phase:

* Independent
* Increased energy level
* Initiates self-care activities
* Assumes increasing responsibility for neonate's care
* Receptive to education for self-care and infant care
* Eager to provide "right" infant care
* Easily loses confidence in ability to care for infant
* Increased focus on infant
* Emotional support required to set realistic goals

### Characteristics of letting-go phase:

* Interdependence between mother and other family members
* Acceptance of real child; gives up fantasy child

* Retains, roles, characteristics and relationships compatible with new role as mother
* Lasts throughout growing years

# Maternal Comfort Measures

## Perineal comfort measures

*Nonpharmacologic therapy*

* Use of ice during first 24 hours
* Heat (whirlpool, sitz bath), 12-24 hours postpartum
* Kegel exercises

*Pharmacologic therapy*

* Administration of analgesic medication (usually oral)
* Application of anesthetic sprays PRN
* Tucks

## Hemorrhoid comfort measures

* Use of ice
* Heat (whirlpool, sitz bath)
* Use of sidelying position
* Tucks

*Pharmacologic therapy*

* Anesthetic ointment or suppository
* Stool softeners
* Avoiding prolonged sitting

**Abdominal comfort measures**

* Lying in prone position
* Ambulation
* Warm bath
* Use of analgesic medication (one hour before breastfeeding for lactating mother to promote comfort)

**Breast engorgement comfort measures**

*Lactating mother*

* Early initiation of breastfeeding
* Supportive bra
* Warm shower
* Warm packs/ice packs

*Nonlactating mother*

* Breast binder/supportive bra
* Ice packs
* Mild analgesic

**Muscular comfort measures**

* Backrubs
* Comfortable positioning
* Warm bath
* Mild analgesic

## Rest measures

* Providing periods of uninterrupted rest
* Transferring telephone calls to nurses station while mother rests

## Sleep measures

* Scheduling maternal assessments during infant feeding times to avoid frequent sleep interruption
* Assisting mother in assuming position of comfort
* Providing backrub
* Relieving sources of discomfort (perineal, abdominal, breast)

## Physiologic well-being measures

* Uterine involution
* Prevention of uterine atony due to distended bladder
* Remind mother to empty bladder often
* Use fundal massage to stimulate uterine contraction
* Administer oxytocin for persistently atonic uterus (to halt excessive blood loss)

## Perineal hygiene

* Changing perineal pad with each voiding
* Use of surgigator with each voiding and bowel movement

* Wiping from front to back after voiding or a bowel movement

**Breast care**

*Nonlactating mother*

* Support bra for first week (bottle-feeding mother)

*Lactating mother*

* Support bra
* Avoiding stimulation of the breast
* Avoiding warm shower water falling directly on breasts
* Use of ice packs to prevent engorgement
* Use of mild analgesia for engorgement discomfort

**Elimination measures**

* Reminding mother to empty bladder often
* Administration of stool softener once or twice daily to promote bowel elimination
* Catheterization if mother is unable to void

**Nutrition measures**

* Adequate fluid intake to support lactation
* Diet which promotes tissue healing
* Bowel elimination
* Sufficient calories

# Maternal Self-Care Measures

## *Perineal self-care*

* Change perineal pad after each voiding or bowel movement
* Wipe from front to back after elimination
* Apply perineal pad to the front first
* Avoid tampons until placental site is healed

## *Breast self-care*

* *Lactating mother*
  * Avoid soap on nipples (causes drying/cracking)
  * Use nonplastic backed breast pads (plastic holds in moisture/causes growth of bacteria)
  * Wear supportive bra
  * Keep nipples dry

* *Nonlactating mother*
  * Supportive bra or breast binder for one week
  * Avoid breast stimulation
  * Complete lactation suppression medication as prescribed

### Post-pain self-care

* Lying in prone position
* Ambulation
* Warm bath
* Use of analgesic medication (one hour before breastfeeding for lactating mother to promote comfort)

### Elimination self-care

* Fluid intake (8-10 glasses of water per day)
* Roughage in diet
* Perineal hygiene information

### Nutrition self-care

* Balanced meals high in protein and Vitamin C to promote tissue healing
* Roughage from fresh fruits and vegetables to prevent constipation

### Rest self-care

* Information about resting or napping in morning and afternoon

### Exercise self-care

* Gradually resuming daily activities
* Performing postpartum exercises as instructed by health care provider

### *Sexual activity self-care*

* Use of nonsexual intercourse intimacy until episiotomy site and placental site have healed

* Placental site is considered healed when lochia discharge has ceased (about 3 weeks)

* Vagina will be dry because of decreased level of estrogen

* Use of water-soluble lubricant will make intercourse more comfortable

* Breastfeeding before sexual intercourse will reduce leaking due to sexual stimulation in lactating mother

### *Immunizations self-care*

* Avoid pregnancy for three months following rubella vaccine

* Need to administer RhoGAM following each birth or abortion for Rh negative mother

## INFANT CARE MEASURES

Educating the parent for infant care involves providing information on and demonstration of daily care activities based on individual parental education needs. Education for the new parents should include the following points:

* Handling (cradle, upright, football hold)
* Positioning (side-lying after feeding)
* Feeding
* Burping

* Nasal and oral suctioning
* Bathing (sponge bath until cord falls off)
* Tub bathing (baby is slippery)
* Umbilical cord care (keep it dry)
* Signs of umbilical cord infection
* Nail care
* Swaddling/wrapping
* Dressing (1 light layer of clothing more than the parent has)
* Taking temperature (axillary preferred)
* Voiding
* Stools (consistency, color, number for breastfed infants)
* Diapering
* Sleep
* Activity
* Crying
* Circumcision care
* Safety (car seat, infant CPR)
* Screening tests
* Immunizations

## Guidelines for Calling Health Care Provider for Infant

* Temperature (100.4 degrees F. axillary; 97.8 degrees F. axillary or less)
* Frequent vomiting over a period of time (6 hours)

* Loss of appetite (refused 2 successive feedings)

* Blue skin color (especially lips)

* Difficult to awaken (lethargy)

* Apnea (15 seconds)

* Bleeding or discharge from any opening

* Diarrhea (2 or more green, watery stools)

* Dehydration (<6 wet diapers in 24 hours, sunken anterior fontanelle)

* Continuous high-pitched cry

## Information for Developmental Adjustment to Parenting Role

* Set priorities for tasks that need to be performed and identify priorities that can wait or can be done by others

* Avoid moving to a new location during the puerperium

* Avoid the temptation to perform exceptional housecleaning (identify housecleaning, cooking, laundry tasks that friends or family can perform)

* Schedule naps (morning and afternoon the first 1-2 weeks; unplug the phone, do not answer the door)

* Go to bed early

* Avoid accepting other responsibilities (care of extended family members, community projects, church activities)

* Schedule quiet time away from the baby and out of the house

* ❋ Schedule "couple time" between mother and father
* ❋ Select contraceptive method before first sexual activity
* ❋ Communicate openly with partner and others
* ❋ Include father in infant care activities
* ❋ Plan for infant day care and return to work
* ❋ Discuss with partner who will do what activities during puerperium and after mother returns to work

## SUMMARY OF METHODS OF CONTRACEPTION

Contraceptives are used to prevent, plan or space pregnancies, to select the number of children desired and to control the timing of the birth of each child. Listed below is a summary of methods available, advantages, disadvantages, side effects and contraindications for each method. Contraceptives are classified as oral contraceptives, spermicides, barrier methods, long-acting methods, voluntary sterilization and fertility awareness methods.

### ORAL CONTRACEPTIVES AVAILABLE IN THE UNITED STATES
**Estimated Estrogen/Progestin Potency**

***Progestin:*** *Intermediate*

***Estrogen:*** *Low*

* Demulen 1/35
* Lo-Ovral
* Levlen
* Nordette

**Progestin**: *Low*
**Estrogen**: *Low*

### Monophasic:

- Brevicon
- Genora 1/35
- Loestrin 1/20
- Loestrin 1.5/30
- N.E.E. 1/35 E
- Nelova 1/35 E
- Norcept-E 1/35
- Ortho-Novum 1/35
- Ovcon-35

- Genora 0.5/35
- Genora 1/35
- Loestrin Fe 1/20
- Modicon
- Nelova 0.5/35 E
- Nelova 1/35 E
- Norethin 1/35 E
- Norinyl 1 + 35

### Biphasic

- Nelova 10/11
- Ortho-Novum 10/11

### Triphasic

- Ortho-Novum
- Tri-Levlen
- Triphasil

- Ortho-Novum7/7/7
- Tri-Norinyl

**Progestin**: *High*
**Estrogen**: *Intermediate*

- Ovral

*Progestin:* *Intermediate*
*Estrogen:* *Intermediate*
  * Demulin 1/50                    * Norlestrin 2.5/50


*Progestin:* *Low*
*Estrogen:* *Intermediate*


### Monophasic
  * Norlestrin 1/50                 * Norlestrin 1/50
  * Ovcon 50


## Achieving Hormonal Balances with Oral Contraceptives

**Side Effects: Estrogen**

*Excess:*
  * Nausea                          * Fluid retention
  * Melasma                         * Hypertension
  * Headache                        * Leukorrhea
  * Breast fullness/tenderness


*Deficiency*
  * Early or midcycle breakthrough bleeding
  * Increased spotting
  * Hypomenorrhea

**Side Effects: Progestin**

*Excess*

- Increased appetite
- Fatigue, feeling tired
- Acne, oily skin
- Depression
- Breast tenderness

- Weight gain
- Hypomenorrhea
- Hair loss, hirsutism
- Monilial vaginitis

*Deficiency*

- Late breakthrough bleeding
- Hypermenorrhea

- Amenorrhea

## ESTROGEN-PROGESTIN CONTRACEPTIVES

*Mode of Action:* **Inhibits ovulation**

*Effectiveness:* **0.1%**

*Advantages:*

- Decreased risk for benign breast cysts and fibroadenomas
- Relief of problems associated with menstrual cycle (cramps, pain)
- Easily reversible
- Prevention of ectopic pregnancy
- Method not associated with intercourse (spontaneity)
- Safety

- Timing of next menses known
- Protection against ovarian and endometrial cancer
- Improvement of acne
- Suppression of functional ovarian cysts
- Protection against acute pelvic inflammatory disease

### Disadvantages:

- Pill must be taken at same time daily
- Side effects
- Decreased effectiveness with other medications (*antibiotics, anticonvulsants*)
- Does not protect against STDs
- Expense
- Does not protect against HIV

### Side Effects:

- Mood changes (in some women)
- Melasma (in some women)
- Circulatory complications (rare)
- Nausea (with first packet or first few pills of each pack)
- Missed menses
- Breast fullness/tenderness (in some women)
- Headaches (in some women)
- Increased risk of liver tumors (rare)
- Spotting or breakthrough bleeding

### Indications:

- Heavy or painful menses
- Recurrent ovarian cysts
- Family history of ovarian cancer
- Patient who desires spacing of pregnancies
- Acne
- Nulliparous women
- Sexually active young women/adolescents
- Nonlactating postpartal women

*Contraindications:*

- Breast cancer
- Diabetes

- Coronary artery disease
- Impaired liver function
- Current or past liver adenoma
- Cholestatic jaundice during pregnancy
- Surgery planned within 4 weeks
- Major surgery (requiring immobilization involving lower extremity)

- Hypertension
- Current or past stroke
- Gallbladder disease
- Heavy smoker
- Past or current thromboembolism
- Sickle cell hemoglobinopathy
- Patient over 50 years age

## PROGESTIN-ONLY CONTRACEPTIVE METHODS
### Implants (norplant); injections
*Mode of Action:* Inhibits ovulation

*Advantages:*

- Highly effective
- Method not associated with intercourse (*spontaneity*)
- No estrogen-related side effects
- Decreased menses, cramping and pain (in some women)

- Easily reversible
- Long-acting (*5 years for implant, 3 months for injection*)
- Scanty or no menses *(in some women)*
- Does not suppress lactation

*Disadvantages:*

- Injections required
- Implant may be slightly visible
- Menstrual cycle disturbance
- Delayed reversal
- High initial expense for implant
- Minor surgery required to insert and remove implant

*Side Effects:*

- Menstrual irregularities
- Bone density decrease
- Breast tenderness
- Interaction with anticonvulsants

*Indications:*

- Continuous contraception
- Long-term spacing of births desired
- Patient does not want sterilization
- Lactation
- Patient does not desire more children
- Side effects have been experienced with other contraception methods

*Contraindications:*

- Acute liver disease
- Unexplained, undiagnosed vaginal bleeding
- Cardiac disease or cerebrovascular disease
- Jaundice
- Thrombophlebitis or pulmonary embolism

## OTHER CONTRACEPTIVE METHODS

*Spermicides:* Chemical which kills sperm

*Advantages:*

- Over-the-counter availability
- Provide lubrication
- Can be used to back up other contraceptive methods
- Easy to apply
- Protection against some STDs
- Temporary method
- Does not interfere with lactation

*Disadvantages:*

- Method associated with intercourse
- Messy
- Typical failure rate of 21%

*Side Effects:*

- Skin irritation in some users

*Indications:*

- Need for back-up method
- Need for method without prescription
- Temporary need

*Contraindications:*

- Vaginal abnormality which prevents correct placement and retention of spermicide in vagina to cover the cervix
- Allergy to ingredients
- Inability to use spermicide correctly

***Barrier Methods:*** Condoms, diaphragm, sponge, cervical cap

***Action:*** Mechanical barrier preventing transportation of the sperm to the ovum

***Advantages:***

- Inexpensive
- Accessible (condoms)
- Safe
- Protection against STDs

***Disadvantages:***

- Method associated with intercourse
- Health provider intervention required (for diaphragm and cap)
- Defective device

***Side Effects:***

- Skin irritation (in some users with some methods)
- Increased risk of urinary tract infections (diaphragm)
- Pap smear abnormalities with cap

***Contraindications:***

- Allergy to rubber, latex, polyurethane or chemicals
- Inability to learn correct insertion/application technique
- History of toxic shock syndrome
- Repeated urinary tract infections

***Intrauterine devices (IUD)***

***Action:*** Not fully understood; may be due to effect on sperm, ova, fertilization, implantation, endometrium and/or fallopian tube

*Advantages:*

- Method not associated with intercourse
- Long-acting contraception
- Easy to use
- Reversible

*Disadvantages:*

- Must be inserted and removed by health provider
- Increased menstrual bleeding (*in some women*)
- Dysmenorrhea (*in some women*)

*Side Effects:*

- Uterine/cervical perforation or embedding (*rare*)
- Expulsion (*during first year in some women*)
- Increased risk for pelvic inflammatory disease (*during first few weeks in some women*)

*Indications:*

- Monogamous relationships
- Multiparous women
- Woman with contraindications to hormonal method

*Contraindications*

- Pregnancy
- PID
- Undiagnosed genital bleeding

**Relative** *(not prescribed unless other methods even less desirable):*

- Purulent cervicitis
- Ectopic pregnancy history
- Undiagnosed irregular bleeding

- Recurrent gonorrhea
- Impaired coagulation
- Postpartal or postabortion infection

- At risk for STD (*multiple partners/partner with multiple partners*)

**Other Relative** *(prescribed with careful monitoring):*

- Valvular heart disease
- Menstrual disorder

- Uterine anomalies
- Anemia

**Sterilization:** Vasectomy (*men*); tubal ligation/blockage (*women*)

**Action:** Prevents ova transport through fallopian tube (*tubal ligation*) and prevents sperm transport through vas deferens (*vasectomy*)

**Advantages:**

- Permanent
- Safe

- Private/Personal

- Highly effective
- Cost effective (over time)
- Not associated with intercourse

**Disadvantages:**

- Minor surgical procedure
- No protection against STDs

- Irreversible

*Indications:*

- Personal preference
- Medical disorders
- Multiparity
- Hereditary disease

*Contraindications:*

- Youth (*under 21 years of age if federal funds involved*)
- Mental incompetence

## Fertility Awareness Methods

*Action:* Abstinence from sexual intercourse during fertile period of menstrual cycle

*Advantages:*

- Safe
- Promote learning about body functions
- No religious objections
- No cost
- Useful to plan pregnancy

*Disadvantages:*

- Extensive abstinence for irregular menstrual cycles
- Extensive counseling to learn correct use of methods

*Side Effects:*

- Frustration during periods of abstinence

*Indications:*

- Personal or religious desire to use "natural" method; willingness to accept unplanned pregnancy

### *Contraindications:*

- Irregular temperature chart results
- Unwillingness to use abstinence during fertile period
- Irregular menstrual cycles
- Anovulatory menstrual cycles
- Inability to keep accurate charts

# CLINICAL VALUES
# AND STANDARDS

# CLINICAL VALUES AND STANDARDS

Standard Laboratory Values ........................................ 167

Laboratory Findings in Pregnancy ........................... 174

High-Risk Population Prenatal
Laboratory Screening ................................................. 177

Fetal Well-Being Screening ......................................... 178

Neonatal Well-Being Screening .................................. 178

Screening for Complications of Childbearing ........... 178

Laboratory Values in the Neonatal Period ............... 179

Common Abbreviations .............................................. 184

Measurement Equivalents .......................................... 192

24-Hour Clock ............................................................ 193

| STANDARD LABORATORY VALUES: PREGNANT AND NONPREGNANT WOMEN | | |
|---|---|---|
| | **PREGNANT** | **NONPREGNANT** |
| **HEMATOLOGIC VALUES** | | |
| Complete Blood Count (CBC)* | | |
| Hemoglobin, g/dl | >11 | 12-16 |
| Hematocrit, PCV, % | >33 | 37-47 |
| Red cell volume, ml | 1500-1900 | 1600 |
| Plasma volume, ml | 3700 | 2400 |
| Red blood cell count, million/$mm^3$ | 5-6.25 | 4-5 |
| White blood cells, total per $mm^3$ | 5,000-15,000 | 5,000-10,000 |
| Polymorphonuclear cells, % | 60-85 | 55-70 |
| Lymphocytes, % | 15-40 | 20-40 |
| Erythrocyte sedimentation rate, mm/h | Elevated second and third trimesters | 20 |

**\* At sea level. Permanent residents of higher levels (e.g. Denver) require higher levels of hemoglobin.**

| STANDARD LABORATORY VALUES: PREGNANT AND NONPREGNANT WOMEN | | |
|---|---|---|
| | **PREGNANT** | **NONPREGNANT** |
| MCHC, g/dl packed RBCs (mean corpuscular-hemoglobin concentration) | No change | 32-36 |
| MCH (mean corpuscular hemoglobin per picogram [less than a nanogram]) | No change | 27-31 |
| MCV/$\mu m^3$ (mean corpuscular volume per cubic micrometer) | No change | 80-95 |
| **Blood coagulation and fibrinolytic activity†** | | |
| **Factors VII, VIII, IX, X** | Increase in pregnancy, return to normal in early puerperium: Factor VIII increases during and immediately after delivery | 50% - 150% of normal |
| **†Pregnancy represents a hypercoagulable state** | | |
| Factors XI, XIII | Decrease in pregnancy | |

| STANDARD LABORATORY VALUES: PREGNANT AND NONPREGNANT WOMEN | | |
|---|---|---|
| | **PREGNANT** | **NONPREGNANT** |
| Prothrombin time (protime) | Slight decrease in pregnancy | 12-14 sec. |
| Partial thromboplastin time (PTT) | Slight decrease in pregnancy and again decrease during second and third stages of labor (indicates clotting at placental site) | 60-70 sec. |
| Bleeding time | No change | 1-3 min (Duke) 2-4 min (Ivy) |
| Coagulation time | No change | 6-10 min (Lee/White) |
| Platelets | No significant change until 3-5 days after delivery, then marked increase (may predispose woman to thrombosis) and gradual return to normal | 150,000 to 400,000/mm$^3$ |

| STANDARD LABORATORY VALUES: PREGNANT AND NONPREGNANT WOMEN | | |
|---|---|---|
| | **PREGNANT** | **NONPREGNANT** |
| Fibrinolytic activity | Decreases in pregnancy, then abrupt return to normal (protection against thromboembolism) | |
| Fibrinogen | 600 mg/dl | 300 mg/dl |
| **MINERAL/VITAMIN CONCENTRATIONS** | | |
| Vitamin $B_{12}$, folic acid, ascorbic acid | Moderate decrease | Normal |
| **SERUM PROTEINS** | | |
| Total, g/dl | 5.5-7.5 | 6-8 |
| Albumin, g/dl | 3.0-5.0 | 3.2-4.5 |
| Globulin, total, g/dl | 3.0-4.0 | 2.3-3.4 |
| **BLOOD SUGAR/ GLUCOSE** (Whole Blood) | | |
| Fasting, mg/dl | $\leq 65$ | 115 |

## STANDARD LABORATORY VALUES: PREGNANT AND NONPREGNANT WOMEN

|  | PREGNANT | NONPREGNANT |
|---|---|---|
| 2-hour postprandial, mg/dl | Under 140 after a 100 g carbohydrate meal is normal | 70-140 |

### CARDIOVASCULAR DETERMINATIONS

|  | PREGNANT | NONPREGNANT |
|---|---|---|
| Blood pressure, mmHg | 120/80* | 90-140/60-90 |
| Pulse, rate/min | 80 | 70 |
| Stroke volume, ml | 75 | 45 ± 12 |

*Value at 20 years of age
*For 30 years of age: 123/82
*For 40 years of age: 126/84

| CARDIOVASCULAR DETERMINATIONS (continued) | | + |
|---|---|---|
| Cardiac output, L/min | 6 | 3.6 |
| Circulation time (arm-tongue), sec | 12-14 | 15-16 |
| Blood Volume, ml | | |
| Whole blood | 5600 | 4000 |
| Plasma | 2400 | 2400 |
| Red blood cells | 1500-1900 | 1600 |

## STANDARD LABORATORY VALUES: PREGNANT AND NONPREGNANT WOMEN

| | PREGNANT | NONPREGNANT |
|---|---|---|
| **CHEST X-RAY STUDIES** | | |
| Transverse diameter of heart | 1-2 cm increase | — |
| Left border of heart | Straightened | — |
| Cardiac volume | 70 ml increase | — |
| **HEPATIC VALUES** | | |
| Bilirubin total | Unchanged | Not more than 1 mg/dl |
| Serum cholesterol | Increase 60% from 16-32 weeks of pregnancy; remains at this level until after delivery | 150-200 mg/dl |
| Serum alkaline phosphate | Increase from week 12 of pregnancy to 6 weeks after delivery | 2-4.5 units (Bodansky) |
| Serum globulin albumin | Increase slight Decrease 3.0 g by late pregnancy | 2.3-3.4 g/dl 3.2-4.5 g/dl |

| STANDARD LABORATORY VALUES: PREGNANT AND NONPREGNANT WOMEN | | |
|---|---|---|
| | **PREGNANT** | **NONPREGNANT** |
| **RENAL VALUES** | | |
| | | |
| Bladder capacity | 1500 ml | 1300 ml |
| Renal plasma flow (RPF), ml/min | Increase by 25%, to 612-875 | 490-700 |
| Glomerular filtration rate (GFR), ml/min | Increase by 50%, to 115-192 | 88-128 |
| Nonprotein nitrogen (NPN), mg/dl | Decreases | 25-40 |
| Blood urea nitrogen (BUN), mg/dl | Decreases | 10-20 |
| Serum creatinine, mg/kg/24 hr | Decreases | 20-22 |
| Serum uric acid, mg/kg/24 hr | Decreases | 250-750 |
| Urine glucose | Present in 20% of gravidas | Negative |

| STANDARD LABORATORY VALUES: PREGNANT AND NONPREGNANT WOMEN | | |
|---|---|---|
| | **PREGNANT** | **NONPREGNANT** |
| Intravenous pyelogram (IVP) | Slight to moderate hydroureter and hydronephrosis; right kidney larger than left kidney | Normal |

| LABORATORY FINDINGS IN PREGNANCY | |
|---|---|
| **Glucose (OHSU norms)** | |
| 1 Hr Screen (50 gram) | < 140 mg/dL |
| 3 Hr GTT (100 grams) | |
|     Fasting | 105 mg/dL |
|     1 Hr | 190 mg/dL |
|     2 Hr | 165 mg/dL |
|     3 Hr | 145 mg/dL |
| * Depending on baseline | |
| WBC x $10^3$: | 5.0 - 15.0 |

## LABORATORY FINDINGS IN PREGNANCY

| | |
|---|---|
| PMN (Neutrophils,"Segs," "Polys") (%) | 60-85 |
| Bands (%) | 0-5 |
| Lymphs (%) | 15-40 |
| Monos (%) | 4-10 |
| Eos (%) | 1-5 |
| Basophils (%) | 0-2 |

## LABORATORY FINDINGS IN PREGNANCY

| Renal Value: | Nonpregnant | Pregnant | PIH |
|---|---|---|---|
| Renal plasma flow | 490-700 ml/min | Increased 25% | Decreased |
| Glomerular filtration rate | 88-128 ml/min | Increased 50% | Decreased |
| BUN | 10-20 mg/dL | Decreased | |
| Serum creatinine | 20-22 mg/kg/24 hrs | Decreased | |
| Serum uric acid | 250-750 mg/kg/24 hrs | Decreased | |
| **Hematologic Values:** | **Nonpregnant** | **Pregnant** | **PIH / HELLP** |
| Thrombocytopenia Hematocrit Platelets | Absent 37-47 % 150,000-350,000/mm$^3$ | Absent > 33% Normal | Present Increased |
| **Liver enzymes:** | | | |
| AST (SGOT) | 7-27 U/L | Normal | Elevated |
| ALT (SGPT) | 1-21 U/L | Normal | Elevated |

## LABORATORY FINDINGS IN PREGNANCY

Shift to left (elevated PMN and bands) =
bacterial infection *if* WBC elevated

If WBC elevated, PMNs and bands are normal,
and lymphs are elevated = viral infection

WBC up to 20,000 are normal in labor
(stress response)

**Chemistry**

| | |
|---|---|
| NA+ | 136-145 mEq/L |
| K+ | 3.5-5.0 mEq/L |
| Cl | 98-106 mEq/L |
| $HCO_3$ | 21-30 mEq/L |

**Iron Indices**:

| | |
|---|---|
| Serum Iron (micro gm/dl) | 40-150 |
| TIBC | 250-400 |
| Transferrin | 200-400 |
| Ferritin ng/ml | 11-122 |

**Folate Indices**:

| | |
|---|---|
| Serum Folate (ng/ml) | 1.8-9.0 |

| | |
|---|---|
| **Vitamin $B_1$ (microgram/dL)** | 5.3-7.9 |
| **Vitamin $B_6$ (ng/ml)** | 25-80 |
| **Vitamin $B_{12}$ (pg/ml)** | 200-1100 |

## LABORATORY FINDINGS IN PREGNANCY

**Liver Function Tests:**

| | |
|---|---|
| AST (SGOT) (U/L) | 7-27 |
| ALT (SGOT) (units/L) | 1-21 |
| LDH (units/L) | 45-90 |
| Bilirubin (mg/L) | < 1.5 |

**Thyroid Function Tests:**

| | |
|---|---|
| Free T. (microgram/dL) | 9.1-14.0 |
| TSH (micro units/m) | < 10 |
| Thyroxine binding ratio | 0.85-1.14 |

Previous use of oral thyroid medicine: order free T4

Enlarged thyroid and/or tachycardia and/or wide diastolic/systolic split: order free T4

Note: 99% of thyroxine is bound to protein; 1% is free and has end-organ effect, tachycardia and/or a wide split diastolic/systolic is found.

### High-Risk Population Prenatal Laboratory Screening

- HIV
- Hepatitis B
- HPV smear
- Renal function tests: (BUN, creatinine, creatinine clearance, electrolytes, total protein excretion)

- Hepatitis A
- Group B streptococci
- Blood smear
- Amniocentesis

## Fetal Well-Being Screening in High-Risk Pregnancy

- Amniocentesis
- Phosphatidylglycerol
- Biophysical Profile
- Chorionic Villus Sampling
- Contraction Stress Test
- Ultrasound
- Creatinine Level
- Nonstress Test
- Percutaneous Umbilical Blood Sampling
- Lecithin/Sphingomyelin Ratio

## Neonatal Well-Being Screening

- Cord Blood pH
- HCT
- Type and Rh
- Glucose
- HGB
- RBC
- Bilirubin

## Screening for Complications of Childbearing

- RBC
- HCT
- Platelets
- Fibrinogen
- Prothrombin
- PTT
- Factors VII, VIII, IX, X
- HGB
- Blood Smear
- Blood Chemistry
- Fibrin Split Products
- PT
- Bleeding Time
- Factors XI, XIII

## Renal Creatinine

- BUN
- Uric Acid
- Creatinine Clearance

## Hepatic Test

- ALT (SGPT)
- AST (SGOT)
- LDH
- Alkaline Phosphatase
- Albumin
- Bilirubin

| LABORATORY VALUES IN THE NEONATAL PERIOD | | | |
|---|---|---|---|
| **Blood Values** | **Term** | **Neonatal** | **Preterm** |
| **Clotting factors:** | | | |
| Activated clotting time (ACT) | | 2 min | |
| Bleeding time (Ivy) | | 2-7 min | |
| Fibrinogen | | 125-300 mg/dl | |
| Hemoglobin (g/dL) | 14.5-22.5 | | 15-17 |
| Hematocrit (%) | 44-72 | | 45-55 |
| Reticulocytes (%) | 0.4-6 | | Up to 10 |

| LABORATORY VALUES IN THE NEONATAL PERIOD | | | |
|---|---|---|---|
| **Blood Values** | Term | Neonatal | Preterm |
| Fetal hemoglobin (% of total) | 40-70 | | 80-90 |
| **Clotting factor:** Nucleated RBC/mm$^3$ (per 100 RBC) | 200 (0.05) | | (0.2) |
| Platelet count/mm$^3$ | 84,000-478,000 | | 120,000-180,000 |
| WBC/mm$^3$ | 9,000-30,000 | | 10,000-20,000 |
| Neutrophils (%) | 54-62 | | 47 |
| Eosinophils and basophils (%) | 1-3 | | |
| Lymphocytes (%) | 25-33 | | 33 |
| Monocytes (%) | 3-7 | | 4 |
| Immature WBC (%) | 10 | | 16 |

## LABORATORY VALUES IN THE NEONATAL PERIOD

| Blood Values | Term | Neonatal | Preterm |
|---|---|---|---|
| **OTHER CHEMISTRY** | | | |
| Bilirubin, direct | | 0-1 mg/dl | |
| Bilirubin, total | | Cord: < 2 mg/dl | |
| Peripheral: Total Bilirubin | | 0-2 days: -6 mg/dl<br>1-2 days: -8 mg/dl<br>3-5 days: -12 mg/dl | |
| **BLOOD GASES** | | | |
| Arterial: | | pH 7.31-7.45 | |
| | | $P_{CO_2}$ 33-48 mmHg | |
| | | $P_{O_2}$ 50-70 mmHg | |
| Venous: | | pH 7.28-7.42 | |
| | | $P_{CO_2}$ 38-52 mmHg | |
| | | $P_{O_2}$ 20-49 mmHg | |
| Alpha-fetoprotein | | 0 | |
| Fibrinogen | | 150-300 mg/dL | |

| **LABORATORY VALUES IN THE NEONATAL PERIOD** | | | |
|---|---|---|---|
| **Blood Values** | **Term** | **Neonatal** | **Preterm** |
| Serum glucose | | 40-60 mg/dL | |
| Urinalysis<br>Volume: 1-7 days, 20-40 ml daily<br>After the 1st week: 200 ml/24 hours<br><br>Ketones: negative<br><br>Protein: negative<br><br>Glucose: negative<br><br>Casts and WBCs: rare<br><br>Osmolarity (mOsm/L): 100-600<br><br>pH: 5-7<br><br>Specific gravity: 1.001-1.018<br><br>Color: clear, straw | | | |

## CARDIOPULMONARY AND RESPIRATORY READINGS

**Blood pressure:**

Term: systolic, 60-80 mmHg; diastolic, 40-50 mmHg

Preterm: systolic, 50-60 mmHg; diastolic, 30 mmHg

Respiratory rate: 30-60 min

Heart rate:  100 bpm (sleeping); 160 bpm (crying)

Baseline: 120-160/min

Tachycardia: ≥ 160 bpm (persistent)

Bradycardia: ≤ 120 bpm (persistent)

## Common Abbreviations In Maternal-Newborn and Women's Health Nursing

| | |
|---|---|
| **ABC** | *Alternative birthing center or airway, breathing, circulation* |
| **AC** | *Abdominal circumference* |
| **ACTH** | *Adrenocorticotrophic hormone* |
| **AFAFP** | *Amniotic fluid alphafetoprotein* |
| **AFI** | *Amniotic fluid index* |
| **AFP** | *α-fetoprotein* |
| **AFV** | *Amniotic fluid volume* |
| **AGA** | *Appropriate for gestational age* |
| **AID or AIH** | *Artificial insemination donor (H designates mate is donor)* |
| **AIDS** | *Acquired Immune Deficiency Syndrome* |
| **ARBOW** | *Artificial rupture of bag of waters* |
| **AROM** | *Artificial rupture of membranes* |
| **BAT** | *Brown adipose tissue (brown fat)* |
| **BBT** | *Basal body temperature* |
| **BL** | *Baseline (fetal heart rate baseline)* |
| **BMR** | *Basal metabolic rate* |
| **BOW** | *Bag of waters* |
| **BP** | *Blood pressure* |
| **BPD** | *Biparietal diameter or bronchopulmonary dysplasia* |
| **BPM** | *Beats per minute* |
| **BSE** | *Breast self-examination* |
| **BSST** | *Breast self-stimulation test* |
| **CC** | *Chest circumference or cord compression* |
| **cc** | *Cubic centimeter* |

| | |
|---|---|
| **CDC** | *Centers for Disease Control* |
| **C-H** | *Crown-to-heel length* |
| **CHF** | *Congestive heart failure* |
| **CID** | *Cytomegalic inclusion disease* |
| **cm** | *Centimeter* |
| **CMV** | *Cytomegalovirus* |
| **CNM** | *Certified nurse-midwife* |
| **CNS** | *Central nervous system* |
| **CPAP** | *Continuous positive airway pressure* |
| **CPD** | *Cephalopelvic disproportion or citrate-phosphate-dextrose* |
| **CPR** | *Cardiopulmonary resuscitation* |
| **CRL** | *Crown-rump length of fetus* |
| **C/S** | *Cesarean section or C-section* |
| **CST** | *Contraction stress test* |
| **CT** | *Computerized tomography* |
| **CVA** | *Costovertebral angle* |
| **CVP** | *Central venous pressure* |
| **CVS** | *Chorionic villus sampling* |
| **D&C** | *Dilation and curettage* |
| **decel** | *Deceleration of fetal heart rate* |
| **DFMR** | *Daily fetal movement response* |
| **DIC** | *Dissemination intravascular coagulation* |
| **dil** | *Dilation* |
| **DM** | *Diabetes mellitus* |
| **DRG** | *Diagnostic related groups* |
| **DTR** | *Deep tendon reflexes* |
| **ECHMO** | *Extracorporal membrane oxygenator* |
| **EDC** | *Estimated date of confinement* |
| **EDD** | *Estimated date of delivery* |

| | |
|---|---|
| **EFM** | *Electronic fetal monitoring* |
| **EFW** | *Estimated fetal weight* |
| **ELF** | *Elective low forceps* |
| **Epis** | *Episiotomy* |
| **FAD** | *Fetal activity diary* |
| **FAS** | *Fetal alcohol syndrome* |
| **FBD** | *Fibrocystic breast disease* |
| **FBM** | *Fetal breathing movements* |
| **FBS** | *Fetal blood sample or fasting blood sugar test* |
| **FECG** | *Fetal electrocardiogram* |
| **FFA** | *Free fatty acids* |
| **FHR** | *Fetal heart rate* |
| **FHT** | *Fetal heart tones* |
| **FL** | *Femur length* |
| **FM** | *Fetal movement* |
| **FMAC** | *Fetal movement acceleration test* |
| **FMD** | *Fetal movement diary* |
| **FPG** | *Fasting plasma glucose test* |
| **FRC** | *Female reproductive cycle* |
| **FSH** | *Follicle-stimulating hormone* |
| **FSHRH** | *Follicle-stimulating hormone releasing hormone* |
| **FSI** | *Foam stability index* |
| **G or grav** | *Gravida* |
| **GDM** | *Gestational diabetes mellitus* |
| **GI** | *Gastrointestinal* |
| **GnRH** | *Gonadotrophin-releasing factor* |
| **GnRH** | *Gonadotrophin-releasing hormone* |

| | |
|---|---|
| **GTPAL** | *Gravida, term, preterm, abortion, living children; a system of recording maternity history* |
| **GYN** | *Gynecology* |
| **HA** | *Head-abdominal ratio* |
| **HAI** | *Hemagglutination-inhibition test* |
| **HC** | *Head compression or head circumference* |
| **hCG** | *Human chorionic gonadotrophin* |
| **hCS** | *Human chorionic somatomammotropin (same as hPL)* |
| **HMD** | *Hyaline membrane disease* |
| **hMG** | *Human menopausal gonadotrophin* |
| **hPL** | *Human placental lactogen* |
| **HVH** | *Herpes virus hominis* |
| **ICS** | *Intercostal space* |
| **IDDM** | *Insulin-dependent diabetes mellitus (Type 1)* |
| **IDM** | *Infant of a diabetic mother* |
| **IGT** | *Impaired glucose tolerance* |
| **IGTT** | *Intravenous glucose tolerance test* |
| **IPG** | *Impedance phlebography* |
| **IUD** | *Intrauterine device* |
| **IUFD** | *Intrauterine fetal death* |
| **IUGR** | *Intrauterine growth retardation* |
| **JCAHO** | *Joint Commission on the Accreditation of Health Care Organizations* |
| **LADA** | *Left-acromion-dorsal-anterior* |
| **LADP** | *Left-acromion-dorsal-posterior* |
| **LBW** | *Low birth weight* |
| **LDR** | *Labor, delivery and recovery room* |

| | |
|---|---|
| **LDRP** | *Labor, deliver, recover, and postpartum in same room* |
| **LGA** | *Large for gestational age* |
| **LH** | *Luteinizing hormone* |
| **LHRH** | *Luteinizing hormone-releasing hormone* |
| **LMA** | *Left-mentum-anterior* |
| **LML** | *Left mediolateral episiotomy* |
| **LMP** | *Last menstrual period or Left-mentum-posterior* |
| **LMT** | *Left-mentum-transverse* |
| **LOA** | *Left-occiput-anterior* |
| **LOF** | *Low outlet forceps* |
| **LOT** | *Left occiput transverse* |
| **L/S** | *Lecithin/sphingomyelin ratio* |
| **LSA** | *Left-sacrum-transverse* |
| **MAS** | *Meconium aspiration syndrome or movement alarm signal* |
| **MCT** | *Medium chain triglycerides* |
| **mec** | *Meconium* |
| **mec st** | *Meconium stain* |
| **M&I** | *Maternity and Infant Care Projects* |
| **ML** | *Midline (episiotomy)* |
| **MLE** | *Midline echo or midline episiotomy* |
| **MRI** | *Magnetic resonance imaging* |
| **MSAFP** | *Maternal serum alpha fetoprotein* |
| **MUGB** | *4-methylumbelliferyl quanidnobenzoate* |
| **multip** | *Multipara* |
| **NANDA** | *North American Nursing Diagnosis Association* |
| **NEC** | *Necrotizing enterocolitis* |
| **NGU** | *Nongonococcal urethritis* |

| | |
|---|---|
| **NP** | *Nurse practitioner* |
| **NPO** | *Nothing by mouth* |
| **NSCST** | *Nipple stimulation contraction stress test* |
| **NST** | *Nonstress test or nonshivering thermogenesis* |
| **NSVD** | *Normal sterile vaginal delivery* |
| **NTD** | *Neural tube defects* |
| **OA** | *Occiput anterior* |
| **OB** | *Obstetrics* |
| **OCT** | *Oxytocin challenge test* |
| **OFC** | *Occipitofrontal circumference* |
| **OGTT** | *Oral glucose tolerance test* |
| **OM** | *Occipitomental (diameter)* |
| **OP** | *Occiput posterior* |
| **p** | *para* |
| **Pap smear** | *Papanicolaou smear* |
| **PBI** | *Protein-bound iodine* |
| **PDA** | *Patent ductus arteriosus* |
| **PEEP** | *Positive end-expiratory pressure* |
| **PG** | *Phosphatidylglycerol or Prostaglandin* |
| **PI** | *Phosphatidylinositol* |
| **PID** | *Pelvic inflammatory disease* |
| **PIH** | *Pregnancy-induced hypertension* |
| **Pit** | *Pitocin* |
| **PKU** | *Phenylketonuria* |
| **PMI** | *Point of maximal impulse* |
| **PPHN** | *Persistent pulmonary hypertension* |
| **Preemie** | *Premature infant* |
| **Primip** | *Primapara* |
| **PROM** | *Premature rupture of membranes* |

| | |
|---|---|
| **PTT** | *Partial thromboplastin test* |
| **PUBS** | *Percutaneous umbilical blood sampling* |
| **RADA** | *Right-acromion-dorsal-anterior* |
| **RADP** | *Right-acromion-dorsal-posterior* |
| **RDA** | *Recommended dietary allowance* |
| **RDS** | *Respiratory distress syndrome* |
| **REEDA** | *Redness, edema, ecchymosis, discharge (or drainage) approximation (a system for recording wound healing)* |
| **REM** | *Rapid eye movements* |
| **RIA** | *Radioimmunoassay* |
| **RLF** | *Retrolental fibroplasia* |
| **RMA** | *Right-mentum-anterior* |
| **RMP** | *Right-mentum-posterior* |
| **RMT** | *Right-mentum-transverse* |
| **ROA** | *Right-occiput-anterior* |
| **ROM** | *Rupture of membranes* |
| **ROP** | *Right-occiput-posterior* |
| **ROP** | *Retinopathy of prematurity* |
| **ROT** | *Right-occiput-transverse* |
| **RRA** | *Radioreceptor assay* |
| **RSA** | *Right-sacrum-anterior* |
| **RSP** | *Right-sacrum-posterior* |
| **RST** | *Right-sacrum-transverse* |
| **SET** | *Surrogate embryo transfer* |
| **SFD** | *Small for dates* |
| **SGA** | *Small for gestational age* |
| **SIDS** | *Sudden infant death syndrome* |
| **SOAP** | *Subjective data, objective data, analysis, plan* |

| SOB | *Suboccipitobregmatic diameter* |
| SMB | *Submentobregmatic diameter* |
| SRBOW | *Spontaneous rupture of the bag of waters* |
| SROM | *Spontaneous rupture of the membranes* |
| STD | *Sexually transmitted disease* |
| STH | *Somatotrophic hormone* |
| STS | *Serologic test for syphilis* |
| SVE | *Sterile vaginal exam* |
| TC | *Thoracic circumference* |
| TCM | *Transcutaneous monitoring* |
| TNZ | *Thermal neutral zone* |
| TSS | *Toxic shock syndrome* |
| U | *Umbilicus* |
| u/a | *Urinalysis* |
| UA | *Uterine activity* |
| UAC | *Umbilical artery catheter* |
| UAU | *Uterine activity units* |
| UC | *Uterine contraction* |
| UPI | *Uteroplacental insufficiency* |
| U/S | *Ultrasound* |
| WBC | *White blood cell* |

## MEASUREMENT EQUIVALENTS

### Metric System

1 Liter (L) =
1,000 milliliters (ml)

1 L. = 1,000 cubic
centimeters (cc)

1 grain (gr) =
60 milligrams (mg)

1 mg = 1,000
micrograms (mcg)

1 gram (G) = 1,000 mg

1 cc = 1 ml

1 ounce (oz) = 30 G

1 ml = 16 minims (m)

2.5 centimeters
(cm) = 1 inch (in)

1 kilogram (kg) =
1,000 G

1 kg = 2.2 pounds (lbs)

1 G = 0.001 kg

15 gr = 1 G

1 mcg = 0.001 mg

### Apothecary

60 grains (gr) = 1 dram

8 drams = 1 ounce

16 ounces = 1 pint (pt)

60 minims = 1 dram

480 minims = 1 ounce

1 dram = 1 tea-
spoon (tsp)

4 drams = 1 tablespoon (tbls)

30 ml = 1 oz

### Household

8 oz = 1 cup

1 teaspoon = 5 ml

1 glass = 240 ml

2 tablespoons = 1 oz

1 quart (qt) = 1,000 ml

1 pint = 500 ml

1 minim = 1 drop (gtt)

1 oz = 30 ml

1 pound = 16 oz

1 gallon = 4 quarts

1 quart = 2 pints

# 24 HOUR CLOCK

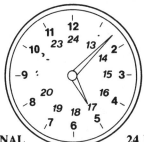

| CONVENTIONAL<br>12 HOUR TIME | 24 HOUR<br>CLOCK TIME |
|---|---|
| 12:01AM | 0001 |
| 1:00 AM | 0100 |
| 1:30 AM | 0130 |
| 2:00 AM | 0200 |
| 3:00 AM | 0300 |
| 4:00 AM | 0400 |
| 5:00 AM | 0500 |
| 6:00 AM | 0600 |
| 7:00 AM | 0700 |
| 8:00 AM | 0800 |
| 9:00 AM | 0900 |
| 10:00 AM | 1000 |
| 11:00 AM | 1100 |
| 12 noon | 1200 |
| 1:00 PM | 1300 |
| 2:00 PM | 1400 |
| 3:00 PM | 1500 |
| 4:00 PM | 1600 |
| 5:00 PM | 1700 |
| 6:00 PM | 1800 |
| 7:00 PM | 1900 |
| 8:00 PM | 2000 |
| 9:00 PM | 2100 |
| 10:00 PM | 2200 |
| 11:00 PM | 2300 |
| 12 midnight | 2400 |

# DRUG
# ADMINISTRATION

# DRUG ADMINISTRATION

Drugs Contraindicated During Breast Feeding......... 197

Medications During Breast Feeding .......................... 197

Commonly Used Medications Containing Aspirin ... 198

FDA Pregnancy Categories ........................................ 199

Commonly Used Medications ..................................... 199

Medications Used in Complications .......................... 213

Toxic Chemical Agents............................................... 230

Nursing Interventions for Emergencies .................... 230

# DRUGS CONTRAINDICATED DURING BREAST FEEDING

- Cocaine
- Diethylstilbestrol
- Cyclophosphamide *(Cytoxan)*
- Ergot
- Gold
- Lithium
- Methadone
- Norethindrone
- Reserpine

- Diazepam *(Valium)*
- Chloramphenicol
- Meprobamate *(Equanil)*
- Ethinyl estradiol
- Heroin
- Marijuana
- Methotrexate
- PCP
- Thiazides

# MEDICATIONS TO USE WITH CAUTION DURING BREAST FEEDING

- Aloe
- Barbiturates
- Depo-Provera
- Dihydrotachysterol
- Indomethacin
- Phenothiazines
- Quinine
- Sulfonamides

- Atropine
- Chloral hydrate
- Dicumarol
- Flagyl
- Isoniazid
- Phenylbutazone
- Senna

## COMMONLY USED MEDICATIONS
## CONTAINING ASPIRIN

- Alka Seltzer
- Alka Seltzer Plus Cold Medicine
- Anacin Maximum Strength
- Arthritis Pain Formula
- Ascriptin
- Axotal
- BAC #3
- BC Powder
- BC Tablets
- Buff-A-Comp
- Buff-A-Comp #3
- Buffaprin
- Bufferin
- Cama Arthritis Strength
- Cope
- Damason-P
- Duradyne
- Empirin #2, #3, #4
- Equagesic
- Equazine-M
- Excedrin
- Fiorinal #1, #2, #3
- Gemnisyn
- Lortab ASA
- Mepro-Analgesic
- Mepro Compound
- Midol
- Midol Maximum Strength for cramps
- Norgesic
- Orphengesic
- P-A-C Tablets
- Rid-A-Pain with Codeine
- Robaxisal
- Soma Compound
- Synalgos DC
- Talwin Compound
- Tecnal
- Trigesic
- Trilisate
- Vanquish

## FDA Pregnancy Categories

**A**   No risk demonstrated to the fetus in any trimester

**B**   No adverse effects in animals, no human studies available

**C**   Only given after risks to fetus are considered: animal studies have shown adverse reactions, no human studies available

**D**   Definite fetal risks, may be given in spite of risks if needed in life-threatening conditions

**X**   Absolute fetal abnormalities; not to be used anytime in pregnancy

## DRUG ADMINISTRATION
## COMMONLY USED MEDICATIONS

**Generic**
*Acetaminophen*

**Classification**
*Non-narcotic analgesic*
*Miscellaneous, antipyretic*

***Pregnancy Category B***

**Trade**

| | |
|---|---|
| Acephen | Neopan |
| Anacin-3 | Panadol |
| Anuphen | Panex |
| APAP | Parcetamol |
| Atasaol | Pedric |
| Banesin | (Robigesic) |
| (Campain) | (Rounax) |
| Datril | St. Joseph's |
| Dolanex | Aspirin-Free |
| Genapap | Suppap |
| Halenol | Tempra |
| Liquiprin | Tenol |
| Myapap | Tylenol |
| N-acetyl-P | Typap |
| aminophenol | Ty-tabs |

**Comments**
*Available:* PO, rectal.
*Used to treat:* Mild to moderate pain, fever.
*Implications:* Assess pain or fever and response to medication. Give with 8 oz. of water. May be given with food or on an empty stomach. Do not give in malnutrition. Tylenol can cause severe liver damage when taken in large amounts over a prolonged period. Use cautiously in pregnancy and lactation. Warn patient against self-medication for more than 10 days (adults) and 5 days (children).
*Common side effects:*
None significant. For overdose, acetylcysteine (mucomyst) is the antidote.

**Generic**
*Butorphanol*

**Trade**
Stadol

**Classification**
*Narcotic Analgesic*
*Agonist/Antagonist*

**Pregnancy Category C**

**Comments**
*Available:* IM, IV.
*Used to treat:* Moderate to severe pain. Used during labor. Also used as a supplement to anesthesia.
*Implications:* Monitor pain relief. Closely monitor vital signs. When used during labor may cause respiratory depression in newborn. Do not use in undiag-

nosed abdominal pain.  Chronic use can cause physical
and psychological dependency.
***Common side effects:***
Sedation, headache, feeling of dysphoria, hypotension,
nausea, diaphoresis.


**Generic**                            **Trade**
*Clindamycin hydrochloride*   Cleocin
                               Dalacin C
**Classification**
*Anti-infective*


***Pregnancy Category B***

**Comments**
***Available:***  PO, IM, IV.
***Used to treat:***  Respiratory tract infections, serious
skin infections, gynecological infections.
***Implications:***  Monitor CBC for decrease in WBC,
platelets.  Monitor for superinfection and signs of
pseudomembranous colitis.  Give PO with full glass of
water.  Give with meals.  Do not refrigerate.  IV:  Do
not bolus undiluted.  1200 mg maximum in single IV infusion.  Do not administer if crystals are present.
***Common side effects:***
Diarrhea, hypotension, phlebitis at IV site.

**Generic**
*Clotrimazole*

**Trade**
Gyne-Lotrimin
Lotrimin
Mycelex

**Classification**
*Antifungal*

***Pregnancy Category B*** (topical, vaginal)
***Pregnancy Category C*** (oral)
**Comments**
***Available:*** PO, topical, vaginal tablets, cream.
***Used to treat:*** Fungal infections, oropharyngeal and vaginal suppositories or cream are used in pregnancy candidiasis.
***Implications:*** Inspect involved skin areas for improvement and increased skin irritation. Use vaginal preparations at bedtime for maximum contact.
***Common side effects:***
Nausea, vomiting, vaginal irritation (with tablets or cream).

**Generic**
*Erythromycin*

**Trade**
E-mycin, Erythromid
Robimycin ophthalmic
     ointment

**Classification**
*Anti-infective*
***Pregnancy Category B***

Ilotycin

**Comments**
***Available:*** PO, IV, topical ophthalmic.
***Used to treat:*** Respiratory infections, streptococcal infections, chlamydia, syphilis, gonorrhea. Primary use

in obstetrics is as prophylaxis for ophthalmia neonatorum.

*Implications:*  Monitor signs of infection, especially temperature.  Crosses placenta and is found in breast milk.  Erythromycin Estolate (estolate salt) is contraindicated in pregnancy.  In the neonate, Ilotycin is used prophylactically for ophthalmic neonatorum, caused by *Neisseria gonorrhoeae* or *Chlamydia* infection acquired from the infected mother during passage through the birth canal.

**Common side effects:**
Nausea, vomiting, diarrhea, abdominal cramping.


| **Generic** | **Trade** |
|---|---|
| *Folic Acid* | Folate |
| | Folvite |

**Classification**
*Vitamin, water soluble*

*Pregnancy Category A*

**Comments**
*Available:*  PO, IM, IV, SC.

*Used to treat:*  Megaloblastic and macrocytic anemias.  Given during pregnancy to enhance normal fetal growth and development.  Stimulates production of RBCs, WBCs, and platelets.

*Implications:*  Monitor folic acid levels, along with hemoglobin, hematocrit, and reticulocyte count.  Crosses the placenta and is found in breast milk.  Administer cautiously in undiagnosed anemias.  Encourage foods high in folic acid:  green leafy vegetables, fruits, organ meats.

*Common side effects:*
Rash, deep yellow urine.

| **Generic** | **Trade** | |
|-------------|-----------|--|
| *Hydroxyzine* | Anxanil | Hydroxacen |
| | Atarax | Hy-Pam |
| **Classification** | Atozine | Vistaril |
| *Sedative-hypnotic* | Durrax | Vistaject-25 |
| *Antihistamine* | E-Vista | Vistaject-50 |

*Pregnancy Category C*

**Comments**
*Available:* PO, IM.
*Used to treat:* Nausea and vomiting, anxiety, severe itching related to allergies and to enhance analyze effect of narcotic. Also used for preoperative sedation.
*Implications:* Contraindicated in early pregnancy but is used during labor. Safety during lactation unknown. Provide for safety as sedation occurs. Give deep, Z-tract if administered IM. Do not use deltoid muscle. Rotate sites if multiple injections given.
*Common side effects:*
Drowsiness, dry mouth, painful IM injection, abscess may occur if not given deep IM.

| **Generic** | **Trade** | |
|-------------|-----------|--|
| *Iron dextran* | Dextraron | Imferon |
| | Feronim | Irodex |
| **Classification** | Hematran | Norferan |
| *Anti-anemic,* | Hydextran | |
| *iron supplement* | | |

### Pregnancy Category B

**Comments**
*Available:* IM, IV.
*Used to treat:* Iron-deficiency anemia.
**Implications**: Give Z-track deep IM into buttocks (never the arm) with a 2-3 inch, 19 or 20 gauge needle. Infuse slowly IV (100 mg over 1-6 hours) or hypotension may occur. Crosses the placenta and is found in breast milk. Do not give oral iron preparations at the same time as parenteral administration.
*Common side effects:*
Hypotension, staining at IM site.

| **Generic** | **Trade** |
|---|---|
| *Methylergonovine* | Methergine |
| | Methylergometrine |

**Classification**
*Oxytocic*

### Pregnancy Category C

**Comments**
*Available:* PO, IM, IV.
*Used to treat:* Or prevent hemorrhage caused by uterine atony; postpartum or post abortion.
*Monitor:* Blood pressure, pulse, uterine contractions; notify physician if contractions do not occur.
*Implications:* Do not administer to induce labor.
Use with extreme caution during third stages of labor.
Found in breast milk, but in small amounts.

*Common side effects:*
Nausea, vomiting, cramping, hypotension, allergic reactions, signs of ergotism: cold extremities, numbness, chest pain, headache, malaise, nausea and vomiting.

| Generic | Trade |
|---------|-------|
| *Metronidazole* | Flagyl |
| | Metizol |
| **Classification** | Protostat |
| *Trichomonacide* | Satric |
| *Amebicide* | |

*Pregnancy Category B*

**Comments**
*Available:* PO, IV, topical.
*Used to treat:* Gynecologic infections, especially trichomoniasis, intra-abdominal infections, bone and joint infections (anaerobic infections).
*Implications:* Monitor closely for super infection. Contraindicated in first trimester. Crosses placenta and is found in breast milk.
*Common side effects:*
Headache, dizziness, nausea and vomiting, abdominal pain, anorexia, diarrhea, superinfection.

**Generic**
*Oxymorphone*

**Trade**
Numorphan

**Classification**
*Narcotic analgesic-agonist*
*Schedule II*

*Pregnancy Category C*

**Comments**
*Available:* SC, IM, IV, rectal.
*Used to treat:* Moderate to severe pain of labor, supplement to anesthesia.
*Implications:* Chronic use in pregnancy and lactation is contraindicated. Crosses the placenta and is found in breast milk, can lead to physical and psychological dependence.
*Common side effects:*
Sedation, confusion, constipation, respiratory depression.

**Generic**
*Oxytocin*

**Trade**
Pitocin
Syntocinon

**Classification**
*Hormone*
*Oxytocic*

*Pregnancy Category C*

**Comments**
*Available:* IV, intranasal.
*Used to facilitate:* Uterine contractions and induction of labor, control postpartal bleeding, as nasal preparation to promote the let down of milk in the lactating woman.
*Implications:* Monitor blood pressure. Use very cautiously in first and second stages of labor, anticipated CS section, and intranasal any time during pregnancy. Assess fetal heart rate, presentation, and gestational age before administration. Monitor uterine contractions and FHR and maternal vital signs throughout administration. For induction of labor administer only as an IV piggyback preferably using an intravenous pump.
*Common side effects:*
Hypotension, painful contractions, signs of water intoxications: headache, confusion, restlessness, anuria.
*Fetus:* Intracranial bleed, hypoxia, dysrhythmias.

| **Generic** | **Trade** |
|---|---|
| *Penicillin* | Bicillin |
| *G. Benzatine* | Bicillin L-A |
| | Permapen |

**Classification**
*Anti-infective*

*Pregnancy Category B*

**Comments**
*Available:* PO, IM.

***Used to treat:*** Wide range of infections, including: pneumococcal pneumonia, streptococcal pharyngitis, syphilis.

***Implications:*** Watch for allergic reaction, obtain C&S cultures before initiating therapy. Give on empty stomach 1 hour before or 2 hours after meals. Use cautiously in pregnancy and lactation. Avoid giving with juice or carbonated drinks. After IM administration, massage well. Crosses the placenta and is found in breast milk.

***Common side effects:***
Nausea, vomiting, diarrhea, epigastric distress, rash, pain IM site.

***Signs of anaphylaxis:*** Rash, itching, wheezing, laryngeal edema.

| **Generic** | **Trade** |
|---|---|
| *Penicillin* | Crystapen |
| *Potassium* | Megacillin |
| | P-50 |
| **Classification** | Nova-Pen G |
| *Anti-infective* | Pentids |
| | Pfizerpen |
| | Pfizerpen G |

***Pregnancy Category B***

**Comments**
***Available:*** PO, IM, IV.
***Used to treat:*** Broad spectrum of infections including pneumococcal pneumonia, streptococcal pharyngitis, syphilis, gonorrhea, Lyme's disease.

*Implications:* Monitor for allergic reaction. Do not give with food, fruit juice or carbonated drinks: obtain C&S cultures before initiating therapy, watch for super-infection. Use cautiously in pregnancy and lactation. Crosses the placenta and is found in breast milk.

**Common side effects:**
Nausea and vomiting, diarrhea, abdominal distress, rash, pain at IM site, phlebitis at IV site, allergic reactions.

**Generic**
*Phytonadione*

**Trade**
AquaMEPHYTON
Vitamin K

**Classification**
*Vitamin*
*Fat Soluble*

*Pregnancy Category C*

**Comments**
*Available:* IM.

*Used to prevent:* Hemorrhagic disease of the new-born.

*Implications:* Carefully monitor for occult bleeding or obvious bleed 2nd or 3rd day of life. Administer: pro-phylactically after birth; protect drug from light.

**Common side effects:**
Rash, pain at injection site, bleeding, allergic reaction.

| Generic | Trade | |
|---------|-------|---|
| *Promethazine* | Anergan 25 | PMS Promethazine |
| | Anergan 50 | Pro-50 |
| **Classification** | (Histantil) | Prometh-25 |
| *Antihistamine* | K-Phen | Prometh-50 |
| *Antiemetic* | Mallergan | Promethegan |
| *Sedative/Hypnotic* | Pentazine | Prorex-25 |
| | Phenameth | Prorex-50 |
| **Pregnancy** | Phenazine 25 | Prothazine Plain |
| **Category C** | Phenazine 50 | V-Gan 25 |
| | Phencen 50 | V-Gan 50 |
| | Phenergan | |
| | Phenergan Fortis | |
| | Phenergan Plain | |
| | Phenoject 50 | |

**Comments**

*Available:* PO, IM, IV, rectal.

*Used to treat:* and prevent nausea and vomiting. Used as an or adjunct to analgesia for labor.

*Implications:* Monitor level of sedation. May cause EPS, usually takes effect within 20 minutes. Administer with food or milk to decrease GI irritation. Used safely during labor, but avoid prolonged use during pregnancy. Use cautiously in lactation. Crosses the placenta.

**Common side effects:**

Sedation, dizziness, hypotension, hypertension, dry mouth, constipation.

*Signs of EPS:* restlessness, twitching, tremors, drooling.

| **Generic** | **Trade** |
|---|---|
| *Rh (D) Immune* | RhoGAM |
| *Globulin* | RhoGAM |
| *Standard Dose* | MICRhoGAM |
| *Rh (D) Globulin* | Mini-Gamulin Rh |
| *MICRODOSE* | |

**Classification**
*Serum immune globulin*

***Pregnancy Category C***

**Comments**
*Available:* IM.
*Used to treat:* Rh negative woman who has delivered
an Rh positive infant, had a miscarriage or abortion,
experienced amniocentesis or other invasive procedure
and prophylactically at 28-30 weeks gestation.
Prevents the production of antibodies in Rh negative
patients and prevents erythroblastosis fetalis (hemolytic
disease) in the newborn in future pregnancies.
*Implications:* Give in deltoid. Do not give IV. Must
be administered within 72 hours of exposure to Rh positive blood and prophylactics at 28 weeks to prevent maternal sensitization. Postpartally type and crossmatch
both the blood of the mother and the newborn to determine need for RhoGAM. Mother must be negative
and infant must be positive.
*Common side effects:*
Fever, painful IM injection.

## MEDICATIONS USED IN
## COMPLICATIONS OF CHILDBEARING

**Generic**
*Betamethasone*

**Trade**
Betnesol
Celestone Phosphate
Cel-U-Jec
Selestoject

**Classification**
*Corticosteroid synthetic*

*Pregnancy Category C*

**Comments**
*Available:* PO, IM, IV.
*Used to treat:* Used to induce pulmonary maturity and reduce incidence of RDS in preterm neonates.
*Implications:* Monitor maternal potassium, blood sugar, urine glucose on long-term therapy; hypokalemia, hyperglycemia.
*Common side effects:*
Maternal acne, poor wound healing, ecchymosis, bruising, depression, flushing, sweating, hypertension, diarrhea, nausea, abdominal distention, increased appetite.

**Generic**
*Cefaclor*

**Trade**
Ceclor

**Classification**
*Antibiotic*

*Pregnancy Category B*

*Comments*
*Available:* PO.

*Used to treat:* Gram-negative bacilli, *H. Influenzae, E. coli, P. Mirabilis, Klebsiella,* gram-positive organisms: *S. Pneumoniae, S. Pyogenes, S. aureus;* upper and lower respiratory tract, urinary tract, skin infections, otitis media.

*Implications:* Assess for sensitivity to penicillins and other cephalosporins, Nephrotoxicity; increased BUN creatinine, I&O, blood studies, electrolytes, bowel pattern qd.

*Common side effects:*
Diarrhea, anorexia, nausea, vomiting, rash.

*Antidote:* Calcium gluconate.

| **Generic** | **Trade** |
|---|---|
| *Cefadroxil* | Duricef |
| | Ultracef |

**Classification**
*Antibiotic*

*Pregnancy Category B*

**Comments**
*Available:* PO.

*Used to treat:* Gram negative bacilli: *E. coli, P. Mirabilis, Klebsiella* (UTI only); gram positive organisms: *S. pneumoniae, S. pyogenes, S. aureus;* upper, lower respiratory tract, urinary tract, skin infections, otitis media, tonsillitis; particularly for UTI.

*Implications:* Assess sensitivity to penicillin or other cephalosporins; nephrotoxicity; increased BUN; I&O daily; blood studies, electrolytes, bowel pattern qd.
*Common side effects:*
Diarrhea, anorexia, nausea, vomiting, rash.
Drugs from the cephalosporins have many of the same side effects and uses. The drug is chosen based on strain of infection, and cost.

| Generic | Trade |
|---|---|
| *Diazepam* | Q-Pam |
| | Stress-Pam |
| **Classification:** | Valium |
| *Antianxiety* | Valrelease |
| | Vasepam |
| | Zetran |

*Pregnancy Category D*

**Comments**
*Available:* Tabs 2, 5, 10 mg; caps ext rel 15 mg, IM/IV inj.
*Used to treat:* Anxiety; seizures.
*Implications:* Assess blood pressure, pulse, respiration; blood studies, hepatic studies (prolonged therapy).
*Common side effects:*
Dizziness, drowsiness, orthostatic hypotension, lethargy.

**Generic**  
*Digitalis glycoside*  
*Digoxin*

**Trade**  
Lanoxin  
Lanoxicaps

**Classification**  
*Cardiac glycoside*  
*Inotropic agent*  
*Anti-arrhythmic*

*Pregnancy Category A*

**Comments**  
*Available:* Caps, Tabs, Elix, Inj.  
*Used to treat:* Congestive heart failure. Increases cardiac output and decreases heart rate.  
*Implications:* Use with caution in pregnancy and lactation (has been used without adverse effects to fetus). Do not give if heart rate is below 60. Do not give with antacids. Crosses placenta and is found in breast milk.  
*Common side effects:*  
Fatigue, bradycardia, nausea, vomiting, anorexia.

**Generic**  
*Furosemide*

**Classification**:  
*Loop diuretic*

**Trade**  
Furoside  
Apo-Furosemide  
Lasix  
Myrosemide

*Pregnancy Category C*

**Comments**
*Available:* Tabs 20, 40 80 mg; oral sol 10 mg/ml, inj. IM, IV 10 mg/ml.
*Used to treat:* Pulmonary edema, edema in CHF, liver disease, hypertension.
*Implications:* Assess hearing, weight loss, I&O daily for fluid loss; rate, depth, rhythm of respirations; effect of exertion; blood pressure lying, standing; postural hypotension; electrolytes; potassium; sodium; chloride glucose in urine of diabetic patient.
*Common side effects:*
Polyuria, hypokalemia, hypochloremia alkalosis, hypovolemia, hypomagnesemia, hyperuricemia, hypocalcemia, nausea, dehydration.

| **Generic** | **Trade** |
|---|---|
| *Gentamicin* | Alcomicin |
| | Cidomycin |
| **Classification** | Garamycin |
| *Antibiotic* | Jenamicin |

*Pregnancy Category C*

**Comments**
*Available:* Inj., IM, IV.
*Used to treat:* Urinary tract infections; bone, skin, and soft tissue infections.
*Implications:* Assess weight before treatment, dosage calculation is based on weight; I&O ratio, daily urinalysis, VS during infusion; IV site for thrombophlebitis including pain, redness, swelling; serum peak, urine pH if used for urinary tract infections.

*Common side effects:*
Nausea, vomiting, anorexia, rash.


**Generic**                          **Trade**
*Heparin*                            Liquaemin
                                     Lipo-hepin

**Classification**
*Anticoagulant*

*Pregnancy Category C*

**Comments**
*Available:* IV, SC.
*Used to treat:* Deep vein thrombosis, pulmonary emboli, prophylaxis of various thromboembolic disorders.
*Implications:* Assess blood, PTT, APTT, ACT, for bleeding and hypersensitivity. Monitor blood pressure for increasing signs of hypertension. Monitor AST and ALT levels.
*Common side effects:*
Bleeding, thrombocytopenia.
*Antidote:* Protamine sulfate.

| Generic | Trade |
|---------|-------|
| *Hydralazine* | Alazine |
| | Apresoline |
| **Classification** | Dralzine |
| *Antihypertensive* | Rolzine |
| *direct-acting peripheral* | |
| *vasodilator* | |

*Pregnancy Category C*

**Comments**
*Available:* PO, IV, IM.
*Used to treat:* Essential hypertension.
*Implications:* Assess BP q 5min x 2hr, q 1hr x 2hr, 4h. Monitor pulse, jugular venous distention, electrolytes, blood studies, potassium, sodium, chloride.
*Common side effects:*
Drug-induced lupus syndrome symptoms, palpitations, reflex tachycardia, angina, shock, headache, tremors, dizziness, anxiety, nausea, vomiting, anorexia, diarrhea.

| Generic | Trade |
|---------|-------|
| *Insulin* | Humulin N |
| *Isophane Suspension NPH* | Iletin II |
| | Insulated NPH |
| **Classification** | Lentard |
| *Exogenous unmodified* | Lente |
| *insulin* | Lente Iletin |
| | Monotard |
| *Pregnancy Catagory B* | Novolin L |
| | Novolin N, NPH |

**Comments**
*Available:* SC, IV.
*Used to treat:* Ketoacidosis, type I (IDDM), type II (NIDDM) diabetes mellitus, Gestational Diabetes.
*Implications:* Assess fasting blood glucose, 2 hr PP. Urine ketones during times of illness, insulin requirements may increase during times of stress, illness, gestation progression in second & third trimesters.
*Common side effects:*
Hypoglycemia, lipodystrophy.

| **Generic** | **Trade** |
|---|---|
| *Insulin, regular* | Humulin BR |
| | Humulin R |
| **Classification** | Iletin I |
| *Exogenous unmodified* | Iletin II |
| *insulin* | Novolin R |
| | Velosulin |

*Pregnancy Category B*

**Comments**
*Available:* IV/SC/inj.
*Used to treat:* Ketoacidosis, type I, II, NIDDM, IDDM, Gestational Diabetes.
*Implications:* Assess for fasting blood glucose, 2 hr PP. Urine ketones during illness, insulin requirements increase during times of stress, illness, gestation progression in second & third trimesters.
*Common side effects:*
Hypoglycemia, lipodystrophy.

**Generic**
*Levothyroxine*

**Classification**
*Thyroid hormone*

**Trade**
Levothroid
Levoxine
Synthroid

*Pregnancy Category A*

**Comments**
*Available:*  PO, IM, IV.
*Used to treat:*  Hypothyroidism, thyroid hormone replacement.
*Implications:*  Assess blood pressure before each dose; I&O ratio, weight qd; pro-time may necessitate decreased anticoagulant.
*Common side effects:*
Irritability, insomnia, nervousness, tachycardia, weight loss.

**Generic**
*Magnesium sulfate*

**Classification**
*Anticonvulsant, Tocolytic*

*Pregnancy Category A*

**Comments**
*Available:*  Inj., IV, IM, 10%, 50%, 12.5%, granules.
*Used to treat:*  Control or prevention of seizures in pregnancy-induced hypertension; treatment of premature labor.

*Implications:* Assess VS, deep tendon reflexes, respirations, urinary output q 15 min after IV dose; do not exceed 150 mg/min; monitor cardiac function; magnesium levels; timing of contractions, determine intensity; fetal heart rate; reactivity may decrease with this drug if used during labor; deep tendon reflexes; respirations; urinary output.

*Common side effects:*

Sweating, depressed deep tendon reflexes, flushing, hypotension, drowsiness, decreased respiratory rate, bradycardia, arrhythmias, hypothermia, oliguria.

*Antidote:* Calcium gluconate.

| Generic | Trade |
|---------|-------|
| *Methyldopa* (Oral)* | Aldomet |
| | Dopamet |
| | Novamedopa |

| Generic | Trade |
|---------|-------|
| *Methyldopate** | Aldomet |
| *Intravenous* | |

**Classification**
*Antihypertensive*

*Pregnancy Category C*

**Comments**
*Available:* PO, IV.
*Used to treat:* High blood pressure by decreasing peripheral resistance.

*Implications:*  Monitor blood pressure and pulse closely.  Use cautiously in pregnancy and lactation. (It has been used safely in pregnancy.)  Crosses placenta and is found in small amounts in breast milk.

**Common side effects:**
Sedation, nasal stuffiness, hypotension, depression, bradycardia, diarrhea.

*Note:  This drug has 2 generic names and two sets of trade names.

| **Generic** | **Trade** |
|---|---|
| *Nifedipine* | Adalat |
| | Apo-Nifed |
| | Novo-Nifedin |
| **Classification** | Procardia |
| *Calcium-channel blocker* | Procardia XL |

*Pregnancy Category C*

**Comments**
*Available:*  PO.
*Used to treat:*  Hypertension (sustained release only) in preeclampsia.
*Implications:*  Monitor cardiac status: blood pressure, pulse, respiration, ECG, urinary output.

**Common side effects:**
Dysrhythmia, nausea, dizziness, lightheadedness, headache, nervousness, dyspnea, cough, wheezing, nasal congestion, sore throat.

**Generic**
*Penicillin G procaine*

**Classification**
*Broad spectrum, long-acting antibiotic*

**Trade**
Crysticillin
Duracillin A.S.
Wycillin
Pfizerpen-AS

*Pregnancy Category B*

**Comments**
*Available:* IM.
*Used to treat:* Gonorrhea, urinary tract infections.
*Implications:* Assess for history of penicillin or cephalosporin reactions, I&O; monitor for hematuria, oliguria; toxicity may occur in patient with compromised renal system. C&S before drug therapy.
*Common side effects:*
Nausea, vomiting, diarrhea, epigastric distress, rash.

**Generic**
*Penicillin G Sodium*

**Classification**
*Broad spectrum antibiotic*

**Trade**
Crystapen

*Pregnancy Category B*

**Comments**
*Available:* IM, IV.
*Used to treat:* Gonorrhea, urinary tract infections.

*Implications:* Assess history of penicillin or cephalosporin reaction. Monitor I&O, hematuria, oliguria; monitor patients with poor renal system; drug is excreted slowly in these patients with poor renal systems. Assess C&S before drug therapy.

**Common side effects:**
Nausea, vomiting, diarrhea, epigastric distress, rash, pain at injection site.

**Generic**
*Propranolol HCl*

**Trade**
Inderal
Inderal LA

**Classification**
*B-Adrenergic blocker*

*Pregnancy Category C*

**Comments**
*Available:* PO.
*Used to treat:* Chronic stable angina pectoris, hypertension, supraventricular dysrhythmias, antidote in tocolytic therapy of ritodrine or terbutaline.
*Implications:* Monitor blood pressure, pulse, respirations during beginning therapy. Report weight of five pounds, monitor I&O ratio. Hepatic, renal function, CBC in prolonged therapy.

**Common side effects:**
Bronchospasm, hypotension, bradycardia, fatigue, weakness, depression, insomnia, diarrhea, nausea, vomiting, Raynaud's phenomenon.

**Generic**
*Propylthiouracil*

**Trade**
Propyl-Thyracil*
PTU

**Classification**
*Thyroid hormone antagonist*

***Pregnancy Category D***

**Comments**
*Available:* PO.
*Used to treat:* Hyperthyroidism, weight loss.
*Implications:* Monitor for hypersensitivity: rash, enlarged cervical nodes, hypoprothrombinemia, bone marrow depression.
*Common side effects:*
Rash, hyperpigmentation, drowsiness, headache, fever, nausea, diarrhea, vomiting.

**Generic**
*Ritodrine HCl*

**Trade**
Yutopar

**Classification**
*Tocolytic uterine relaxant*

***Pregnancy Category B***

**Comments**
*Available:* PO, IV.
*Used to treat:* Pre-term labor.
*Implications:* Assess for maternal, fetal heart tones during infusion; intensity length of uterine contractions;

fluid intake to prevent fluid overload; monitor blood glucose in diabetics.

**Common side effects:**
Hyperventilation, headache, widening pulse pressure, restlessness, anxiety, nervousness, sweating, nausea, vomiting, anorexia, hypoglycemia, hypokalemia.

| **Generic** | **Trade** |
|---|---|
| *Sodium bicarbonate* | Bell-ans |
| | Citrocarbonate |
| **Classification** | Neut |
| *Alkalizer* | |

**Pregnancy Category C**

**Comments**
*Available:* PO, IV.
*Used to treat:* Metabolic acidosis, cardiac arrest, alkalization (systemic/urinary).
*Implications:* Monitor respiratory rate and pulse rate, rhythm, depth, lung sounds, FHR; Assess for edema, I&O, urine pH; monitor electrolytes, blood pH, Pos, HCO3 during treatment, ABGs during emergency situations.

**Common side effects:**
Twitching, hyperreflexia, belching, gastric distention, alkalosis.

**Generic**
*Sulfadiazine*

**Classification**
*Antibiotic*

*Pregnancy Category C*

**Comments**
*Available:* Tabs 500 mg.
*Used to treat:* Urinary tract infections, chancroid.
*Implications:* I&O ratio; color, character, pH of
urine. Monitor for desired output of 800 ml less than
intake. Administer on an empty stomach; ensure adequate water intake (drug is very insoluble and may
cause crystalluria if high concentration occurs).
*Common side effects:*
Nausea, vomiting, abdominal pain, headache, photosensitivity.

**Generic**
*Sulfamethizole*

**Trade**
Sulfasol
Thiosulfil

**Classification**
*Antibiotic*

*Pregnancy Category C*

**Comments**
*Available:* PO.
*Used to treat:* Urinary tract infections.

*Implications:* Assess I&O, note color, character of urine; assess for desired output of 800 ml less than intake. C&S before beginning therapy, administer on an empty stomach, ensure adequate fluid intake (drug very insoluble).

**Common side effects:**
Nausea, vomiting, abdominal pain, headache, photosensitivity.

**Generic**
*Terbutaline sulfate*

**Classification**
*Selective B₂-agonist*
*Tocolytic*

**Trade**
Brethaire
Brethine
Bricanyl

*Pregnancy Category B*

**Comments**
*Available:* PO, IV.
*Used to treat:* Bronchospasm, premature labor.
*Implications:* Assess BP, pulse, FHR, uterine contractions.
**Common side effects:**
Tremors, tachycardia, palpitations, tremor, anxiety, headache, hypoglycemia.
*Antidote:* Inderal.

## Toxic Chemical Agents

- Alcohol
- Chemotherapeutic agents
- Chloroquine
- Carbon monoxide
- Coumarins
- Lead
- LSD
- Methamphetamine
- Salicylates
- Tetracycline
- Arsenic
- Barbiturates
- Cigarette smoking
- Cocaine
- Heroine
- Lithium carbonate
- Mercury
- Radiation
- Streptomycin
- Thalidomide

## Nursing Interventions Used in Obstetric Emergencies

### Prenatal Hemorrhage

- Whole blood
- Packed RBCs

### Postpartal Hemorrhage

- Fresh frozen plasma with platelets
- Oxytocin
- Blood
- Methergine (methylergonovine)
- Prostaglandin F2a

### Severe PIH and Eclampsia

- Magnesium sulfate
- Valium (diazepam)
- Phenobarbital sodium

# NURSING CARE
# PLANNING

# NURSING CARE PLANNING

The Nursing Process ..................................................... 233

The Nursing Process in Action ................................. 234

Guidelines for Therapeutic Communication .............. 236

Barriers to Therapeutic Communication ................... 238

Documentation: The Vital Link to
Communication ......................................................... 239

What To Chart ............................................................ 239

How to Chart ............................................................. 241

Protecting Yourself Legally ....................................... 242

More Guidelines to Prevent Malpractice ................... 243

# THE NURSING PROCESS

The term "Nursing Process" was first used in 1955 and since then has become the hallmark of quality nursing care. The nursing process is a systematic, cyclic process which evolves into five steps that emphasize individualized care. Nurses are charged with the accountability of implementing the nursing process.

The five steps of the nursing process are assessment, nursing diagnosis, planning or outcome criteria, intervention, and evaluation. Each part of the process has its specific criteria for nursing action:

1. Assessing the patient's condition.

2. Identifying and stating the problem with a nursing diagnosis.

3. Planning priorities of care with specific outcome criteria.

4. Intervening to effectively implement that plan.

5. Evaluating the patient's response and outcome based upon outcome criteria.

The nursing process begins with the interview and history. When the assessment is complete, a nursing diagnosis is made, patient goals are set, outcome criteria for evaluation are determined and nursing interventions are ordered. Once this cycle is completed, reassessment is necessary. The nurse explores why and how the plan of care did or did not work.

Assessment and nursing diagnoses are the foundation of the nursing process and the nursing plan of care. In order to effectively utilize nursing diagnoses, it is important to understand the three components of a nurs-

ing diagnosis, all of which must be documented. They
are:

- Statement of the problem. Identifying conditions
  from the NANDA list of nursing diagnoses that
  address independent nursing care.

- Etiology of the problem: Identifying the probable
  cause of a patient's problem or potential problem.

Defining characteristics of the problem. Selecting the
specific objective and subjective data gathered during
the assessment that relate to this particular problem.
Each component of the nursing process along with a
specific design resulting in specific nursing actions is
summarized in the following table.

## THE NURSING PROCESS IN ACTION

### *THE PROCESS*

*Assessment*

### *THE DESIGN*

- Collect, verify and organize the data. Recog-
  nize problems and potential problems. Ask the
  question: "What's going on with this patient in
  this situation?"

### *THE ACTION*

*Interview*

- Patient history
- Physical exam
- Lab data

- Physician's history
- Systems assessment

## THE PROCESS

*Nursing diagnosis*

- Specifically identify and label problems and potential problems. Ask the question, "What is the problem and the potential problem in this situation?"

## THE ACTION

*Analyze data*

- Derive nursing diagnosis from the NANDA list. Establish the priority of problems identified.

## THE PROCESS

*Planning/Outcome criteria*

- Plan priorities of care that are realistic for that individual. Patient-oriented goals, called outcome criteria, must be measurable and specific. These criteria are the basis upon which evaluation will be made. Ask the question, "What can the patient accomplish in this situation?"

## THE ACTION

- Determine what the patient is able to achieve and ask the patient for input in the plan of care. Give the patient as much control as possible. Delegate action and decide upon the focus of decision.

## THE PROCESS

*Intervention*

- What will the nurse do to help the patient accomplish planning/outcome goals? Determine what the dependent interventions and independent interventions will be. Ask the question, "What can I do to help the patient in this situation?"

## *THE ACTION*

- Perform nursing interventions. Begin reassessing what works and what does not. Be sure to intervene based on scientific rationales whether they are actually written on the plan of care or not.

## *THE PROCESS*

*Evaluation*

- Determine to what extent goals have been achieved. Assess patient response. Evaluate progress based upon outcome criteria. Ask the question, "Is the patient better or worse? Why?"

## *THE ACTION*

- Compare patient response to outcome criteria. Analyze why the patient responded the way he did. Reassess. Update plan of care. Ask the question, "What do we do now?"

## GUIDELINES FOR THERAPEUTIC COMMUNICATION IN A HELPING RELATIONSHIP

* Be congruent in what you are saying and what your body language is conveying.

* Use clear, concise words that are adapted to the individual's intelligence and experience.

* Do not say, "I understand." Nonverbally or verbally say, "I care about you."

* Use appropriate silence to give the patient time to organize his thoughts.

* Let the patient set the pace of the exchange—do not hurry him.

* Accept the patient as he is.  The nursing profession espouses empathy without judgment.

* Offer a collaborative relationship in which you are willing to work with the patient in resolving problems but not to resolve these problems for him.

* Use open-ended questions to encourage expression of feelings and ideas.

* Explore ideas completely.  Do not drop a subject that the patient has brought up without some resolution.

* Clarify statements and relationships when necessary.  Do not try to read the patient's mind.

* Give positive feedback every chance you get.  Praise the patient for communication and attempts at problem-solving.

* Encourage expression of feelings.

* Paraphrase statements and feelings to facilitate further talking.

* Translate feelings into words so that hidden meanings can be discovered.

* Focus on reality, especially if the patient misinterprets the facts or if he is misrepresenting the truth.

* Offer teaching and information, but avoid giving advice.

* Search for mutual, intuitive understanding.  Encourage the patient to ask for clarification if he does not understand what is being said.  Do not use slang or phrases that can be misunderstood.

* Encourage an appropriate plan of action, such as problem-solving or self-care.

* Summarize at the end of the conversation to focus on the important points of the communication and validate the patient's understanding.

* Remember, the more personal and intense a feeling or thought is, the more difficult it is to communicate. Give the patient the time and the security to express his deepest feelings. The key word is *listen*.

## BARRIERS TO THERAPEUTIC COMMUNICATION

Therapeutic communication techniques are valuable. However, the attitude of caring is the foundation of therapeutic transaction. The nurse should be aware of actions that often block communication.

- Using words that the patient does not understand or inappropriate cliches.

- Inferring to the patient that you are in a hurry or preoccupied with other tasks.

- Showing anger or anxiety, especially when those feelings provoke an argument with the patient.

- Incorrectly interpreting what the patient expresses.

- Offering counseling when the timing is wrong or when the patient is not ready to hear what is being communicated.

- Giving false reassurance and discounting the patient's feelings.

- Expressing opinions and giving advice, especially when these feelings provoke an argument with the patient.

- Persistently asking probing questions that make the patient uncomfortable.
- Being insincere. (Patients pick this up very quickly.)
- Interrupting while the patient is talking.

## DOCUMENTATION—THE VITAL LINK TO COMMUNICATION

The purpose of charting is to communicate the care given to the patient. Documentation of nursing care must be as complete and congruent as the care itself. Documentation is the best way for a nurse to provide accountability in situations where she is responsible for patient care. The battle cry on the documentation front has become: "If it is not charted, it is not done."

## WHAT TO CHART

The Head-to-Toe Systems Assessment. Get a general impression of what is going on with the patient, then focus on particular problems. Carefully assess the situation by asking yourself:

What do I see? _____

What do I hear? _____

What do I think? _____

What will I do? _____

What should I do? _____

What has already been done? _____

How is the patient responding? _____

The nursing process must be charted each shift by recording a nursing physical assessment, nursing diagnoses based on problems and potential problems, goals of patient care, nursing interventions and an evaluation of the patient's progress.

- Any change in conditions, especially if the patient's condition is deteriorating.
- Be as specific as possible, using descriptive details rather than conveying a judgmental tone.
- Include patient response to any treatment or medication.
- Describe patient's understanding of any health teaching.
- Show continuity of care, especially with treatments that require frequent monitoring, such as IV therapy.
- Patient's medical diagnosis and treatments should be noted at least once each shift.
- Indicate all contacts with the physician, including details and direct quotes when pertinent.
- Chart exact times of patient activities, treatments or procedures.
- Chart patient care at least every two hours.
- Correlate documentation regarding the nursing care plan, physician's orders and treatment plan.

## HOW TO CHART

- Always chart in the correct color of ink.
- Write legibly using accurate and concise medical terminology.
- Spell correctly.
- Addressograph and date must be on each page.
- Do not skip lines.
- Do not write between the lines.
- Do not skip times—chart in a time sequence.
- Chart at least every two hours.
- Do not chart in advance of nursing care administered.
- Close entries with name and title.
- Designate late entries as LATE ENTRY with the time.
- Make one line through an error, write ERROR, and sign.
- Never erase.  Never use liquid cover-up or erasable pens.
- If  page must be recopied, draw a single diagonal line across the original and designate book "copy" and original on the appropriate page.
- Do not chart for anyone else; never let anyone else chart for you.
- Use only those abbreviations accepted by your agency.
- Use direct quotes when appropriate.
- Be objective.  Do not draw conclusions or write judgments.

- Avoid such words as "good," "normal" and "appears to be."
- The more descriptive the details, the better.

## PROTECTING YOURSELF LEGALLY

- There are two key elements in protecting yourself legally— documentation and respect for the patient and family. A patient who is shown respect rarely sues. However, adequate documentation is the surefire defense when a nurse is required to prove accountability.
- Complete documentation will safeguard the nurse if she becomes involved in a lawsuit. The nursing notes should reflect that the nurse practiced reasonable and prudent care under the circumstances.
- Biased feelings and judgmental thoughts should never be included in the nursing notes on the chart. Nurses should avoid the use of words such as "uncooperative" and "hostile." When these actions are recorded, they should be written as a fact using direct quotes.
- It is important that you always document that you are following the policy and procedure of the hospital. If you catheterize a patient, note that it was done by sterile technique. If you change IV tubing and the policy and procedure states that it should be done every 48 hours, make a note that this was done. Every small detail of the policy and procedure does not need to be cited. However, it should be noted that a special procedure was done according to policy and procedure.

- There are many reasons the nurse should know the policy and procedure of the hospital where she works. If there is a necessity for a particular policy, then it is important. Legally, it is of utmost importance to follow policy and procedure because if a nurse is involved in an incident, and she did not follow policy and procedure, the hospital malpractice is not obligated to defend her. When this happens, the nurse must supply her own defense. This is one reason that it is a good idea to carry private malpractice insurance.
- It is essential to document any procedure that involves the patient. If it is not charted on the medical record, legally it is not done.

## MORE GUIDELINES TO PREVENT MALPRACTICE

Always exercise reasonable and prudent care under the circumstances.

- Be thoroughly knowledgeable of the hospital's policy and procedure.
- Show concern and caring about your patient.
- Show positive regard to the family. Research indicates family members are more likely to sue than the patient.
- Keep your nursing knowledge current.
- Stay knowledgeable about nursing standards of care.

- Keep current by reading nursing journals on a regular basis.
- Be selective in delegating nursing responsibilities.
- Complete charts in a timely manner.
- Always be aware of the patient's safety.
- Exercise precaution in administering medications.

# PROFESSIONAL
# NETWORK

# PROFESSIONAL NETWORK

How to Write a Resume.............................................. 247

Guidelines to a Successful Job Interview................... 249

Boards of Nursing By State....................................... 250

State Nurses Associations.......................................... 261

Nurses Organizations................................................. 266

Resources for Maternal Care Nurses........................ 269

Professional Organizations........................................ 273

Public Health Organizations ..................................... 274

Sex Education and Therapy....................................... 274

Sexually-Transmitted Diseases .................................. 275

# HOW TO WRITE A RESUME

A resume should be concisely written and organized for at-a-glance reading. Employers quickly screen resumes, and they are often the basis for that important first impression. A professional resume consists of seven components.

I. **The Cover Letter**

   - Use an appropriate business letter format.
   - State the reason you are applying for the position.
   - Emphasize how your qualifications meet their requirements.
   - Request to schedule an interview.
   - State that you have enclosed your resume.

II. **Personal Data**

   - Name
   - Address/telephone number
   - Professional license number
   - Social security number
   - Sex
   - Age
   - Race

### III.  Job Objectives
- Type of position you are seeking
- How your abilities and skills qualify you for this position

### IV.  Educational Background
- Where and when you went to school
- Degrees earned
- Continuing education courses taken

### V.   Work Experience
- Place and dates of employment, beginning with present. Include volunteer work when applicable
- Concisely emphasize major work responsibilities

### VI.  Extracurricular Activities
- Personal development
- Hobbies
- Professional organizations

### VII.  References
Names and addresses of three persons. Include one personal and two professional references. Avoid the names of relatives.

## GUIDELINES TO A SUCCESSFUL JOB INTERVIEW

What will the interviewer ask? The following are broad statements that will cover inquiries during the interview.

- Tell about yourself. Briefly and concisely outline your strengths. Concentrate on your professional, not personal, accomplishments.
- Tell about your qualifications for the job.
- List your strongest and most recent qualifications. Tell why you want the job. Know something about the employer. Be able to say something positive about the company. Avoid using money as a reason.
- Never be critical about past employers, especially if you are changing jobs. Avoid negative comments throughout the interview.
- Tell about your ambitions. Mention that you look forward to new challenges and responsibilities.
- Mention strengths in regard to your new position.
- Mention weaknesses or problems that have been good experiences for you.
- Tell about your salary requirements. Give a range based on an annual wage. De-emphasize money as your motivation for wanting the job.

# BOARDS OF NURSING BY STATE

The following is a list of the state boards of nursing and continuing education requirements for each state

| State | Board of Nursing | CE Requirements |
|---|---|---|
| Alabama | Board of Nursing<br>PO Box 303900<br>Montgomery, AL 36130<br>(205) 242-4360 | 24 hours<br>every 2 years<br>beginning in<br>1993 |
| Alaska | Board of Nursing<br>3601 C. Street, Suite 722<br>Anchorage, AK 99503<br>(907) 269-8161 | 30 contact<br>hours in 2<br>years for<br>nurse<br>practitioners |
| Arizona | Board of Nursing<br>1651 E. Morten, Ste. 150<br>Phoenix, AZ 85020<br>(602) 255-5092 | None |
| Arkansas | State Board of Nursing<br>1123 South University<br>Suite 800<br>Little Rock, AR 72204<br>(501) 686-2700 | None |
| California | Board of Nursing<br>Box 944210<br>Sacramento, CA<br>94244-2100<br>(916) 322-3350 | 30 contact<br>hours every<br>2 years |

| Colorado | Board of Nursing<br>1560 Broadway<br>Suite 670<br>Denver, CO  80202<br>(303) 894-2430 | 20 contact<br>hours every<br>2 years |
|---|---|---|
| Connecticut | Board of Nursing<br>410 Capitol Ave.<br>MS #12 NUR<br>PO Box 340308<br>Hartford, CT 06134<br>(860) 509-7624 | None |
| Delaware | Board of Nursing<br>Cannon Building, Ste. 203<br>Box 1041<br>Dover, DE  19903<br>(302) 739-4522 | 30 contact<br>hours every<br>2 years |
| District of<br>Columbia | Nurses Examining Board<br>614 H Street, N.W.<br>Room 112<br>Washington, D.C. 20001<br>(202) 727-7468 | None |
| Florida | Board of Nursing<br>4080 Woodcock Dr.<br>Suite 202<br>Jacksonville, FL 32207<br>(904) 858-6940 | 24  contact<br>hours every 2<br>years |

| | | |
|---|---|---|
| Georgia | Board of Nursing<br>166 Pryor Street, S.W.<br>Suite 400<br>Atlanta, GA 30303<br>(404) 656-3943 | None |
| Hawaii | Board of Nursing<br>Box 3469<br>Honolulu, HI 96801<br>(808) 586-2695 | None |
| Idaho | Board of Nursing<br>PO Box 83720<br>Boise, ID 83720<br>(208) 334-3110 | Nurse practi-<br>tioners 60<br>contact<br>hours every<br>2 years |
| Illinois | Department of Profes-<br>sional Regulation<br>100 West Randolph<br>Ste. 9-300<br>Chicago, IL 60601<br>(312) 814-2715 | None |
| Indiana | Board of Nurses<br>Registration<br>402 W. Washington St.<br>Suite 041<br>Indianapolis, IN 46204<br>(317) 232-2960 | None |

| | | |
|---|---|---|
| Iowa | Board of Nursing<br>State Capitol Complex<br>1223 E. Court Avenue<br>Des Moines, IA 50319<br>(515) 281-3255 | 45 contact<br>hours every<br>3 years |
| Kansas | Board of Nursing<br>Landon State Office Bldg.<br>Suite 551-5<br>900 S.W. Jackson<br>Topeka, KS 66612<br>(913) 296-4929 | 30 contact<br>hours every<br>2 years |
| Kentucky | Board of Nursing<br>312 Wittington Parkway<br>Suite 300<br>Louisville, KY 40222<br>(502) 329-7000 | 30 contact<br>hours every<br>2 years, in-<br>cluding 2<br>hours of<br>HIV/AIDS<br>education |
| Lousiana | Board of Nursing<br>3510 N. Causeway Blvd.<br>Ste. 501<br>Metairie, LA 70002<br>(504) 568-5464 | 30 contact<br>hours every<br>2 years, or<br>20 hours<br>plus 320<br>hours active<br>practice |
| Maine | Board of Nursing<br>State House Station #158<br>Augusta, ME 04333<br>(207) 624-5275 | None |

| Maryland | Board of Nursing<br>4140 Patterson Ave.<br>Baltimore, MD 21215<br>(410) 764-5124 | None |
| Massachusetts | Board of Registration<br>in Nursing<br>Leverett Saltonstall Bldg.<br>Room 1519<br>100 Cambridge Street<br>Boston, MA 02202<br>(617) 727-9961 | 15 contact<br>hours every<br>2 years |
| Michigan | Board of Nursing<br>Michigan Dept of Commerce<br>Ottawa Towers N.<br>611 W. Ottawa<br>Lansing, MI 48933<br>(517) 373-1600 | None |
| Minnesota | Board of Nursing<br>2700 University Avenue<br>West # 108<br>Saint Paul, MN 55114<br>(612) 642-0567 | 30 contact<br>hours every<br>2 years |
| Mississippi | Board of Nursing<br>239 N. Lamar<br>Ste. 401<br>Jackson, MS 39201<br>(601) 359-6170 | Nurse practi-<br>tioners 40<br>hours every<br>2 years |

| Missouri | Board of Nursing<br>Box 656<br>3523 N. Ten Mile Drive<br>Jefferson City, MO 65102<br>(573) 751-0681 | None |
| --- | --- | --- |
| Montana | Board of Nursing<br>111 North Jackson<br>PO Box 200513<br>Helena, MT 59620<br>(406) 444-2071 | None |
| Nebraska | Nebraska Department<br>of Health<br>P.O. Box 95007<br>Lincoln, NE 68509<br>(402) 471-2115 | 20 contact hours and 200 hours of nursing practice every 5 years, or 75 contact hours |
| Nevada | Board of Nursing<br>PO Box 46886<br>Las Vegas, NV 89114<br>(702) 739-1575 | 30 contact hours every 2 years |
| New Hampshire | Board of Nursing<br>Health and Welfare Bldg.<br>6 Hazen Dr.<br>Concord, N H 03301<br>(603) 271-2323 | Nurse practitioners 20 hours every 2 years |

| | | |
|---|---|---|
| New Jersey | Board of Nursing<br>PO Box 45010<br>Newark, N J 07101<br>(201) 504-6493 | None |
| New Mexico | Board of Nursing<br>4206 Louisiana Blvd., NE<br>Suite A<br>Albuquerque, NM 87109<br>(505) 841-8340 | 30 hours<br>every 2<br>years; 50<br>hours for<br>nurse practi-<br>tioners |
| New York | Board of Nursing<br>State Education Department<br>Cultural Education Center<br>Room 3023<br>Albany, N Y 12230<br>(518) 474-3843 | None |
| North<br>Carolina | Board of Nursing<br>P.O. Box 2129<br>Raleigh, NC 27602<br>(919) 782-3211 | None |
| North Dakota | Board of Nursing<br>919 S. 7th St.<br>Ste. 504<br>Bismark, ND 58504<br>(701) 328-9777 | |

| Ohio | Board  of Nursing<br>77 High St.<br>17th Floor<br>Columbus, OH 43266<br>(614) 466-3947 | None |
| --- | --- | --- |
| Oklahoma | Board of Nursing<br>2915 North Classen Blvd.,<br>Suite 524<br>Oklahoma City, OK 73106<br>(405) 525-2076 | None |
| Oregon | Board of Nursing<br>800 N.E. Oregon St.<br>Box 25, Ste. 465<br>Portland, OR  97005<br>(503) 731-4745 | Nurse practi-<br>tioners 100<br>contact<br>hours every<br>2 years |
| Pennsylvania | State Board of Nursing<br>P.O. Box 2649<br>Harrisburg,  PA<br> 17105-2649<br>(717) 783-7142 | None |
| Rhode Island | Board of Nursing<br>Professional  Regulation<br>3 Capitol Hill, Room 104<br>Providence, RI    02908<br>(401) 277-2827 | None |

| South Carolina | Board of Nursing<br>220 Executive Center Drive<br>Ste. 220<br>Columbia, S C 29210-8420<br>(803) 731-1648 | None |
|---|---|---|
| South Dakota | Board of Nursing<br>3307 South Lincoln Ave.<br>Sioux Falls, SD 57105-5224<br>(605) 367-5940<br>Fax: (605) 367-5945 | None |
| Tennessee | Board of Nursing<br>283 Plus Park Blvd<br>Nashville, TN 37129-5407<br>(615) 367-6232 | None |
| Texas | Board of Nurse Examiners<br>1901 Burnet Road,<br>Suite 104<br>Austin, Texas 78758<br>or (mailing address)<br>Box 140466<br>Austin, TX 78714<br>(512) 305-7400 | 20 contact hours every 2 years |
| Utah | Department of Commerce<br>Division of Occupational<br>and Professional Licensing<br>PO Box 45805<br>Salt Lake City, UT 84145-0805<br>(801) 530-6628 | Must work 1200 hours |

| Vermont | Board of Nursing<br>109 State Street<br>Montpelier, VT 05609<br>In Vermont:<br>(800) 439-8683<br>Outside: (802) 828-2396 | CEU : None<br>Practice re-<br>quirements:<br>400 hours in<br>2 years or<br>960 hours in<br>5 years |
|---|---|---|
| Virginia | Board of Nursing<br>6606 W. Broad St.<br>4th Floor<br>Richmond, VA  23230<br>(804) 662-9909 | None |
| Washington | Board of Nursing Care<br>Quality Assurance Commission<br>Box  47864<br>Olympia, WA  98504<br>(206) 753-2686 | None |
| West Virginia | Board of Examiners for<br>Registered Professional Nurses,<br>101 Dee Dr.<br>Charleston, WV  25311<br>(304) 558-3596 | None |
| Wisconsin | Department of<br>Regulation and Licensing<br>Board of Nursing<br>1400 E. Washington Ave.<br>Madison, WI  53708<br>(608) 267-2357 | None |

| Wyoming | State Board of Nursing<br>2020 Carey Ave.<br>Ste. 110<br>Cheyenne, WY 82002<br>(307) 777-7601 | 20 hours in 2 years or practice for 500 hours in 2 years or 1600 hours in 5 years or pass RN NCLEX within last 5 years |

# STATE NURSES ASSOCIATIONS

The American Nurses Association is supported by the following 53 state organizations.

Alabama State
Nurses Association
360 North Hull Street
Montgomery, AL 36104-3658
(205) 262-8321

Alaska Nurses
Association
237 East Third Avenue
Anchorage, AK 99501
(907) 274-0827

Arizona Nurses Association
1850 East Southern Avenue,
Suite 1
Tempe, AZ 85282
(602) 831-0404

Arkansas State Nurses
Association
117 South Cedar Street
Little Rock, AR 72205
(501) 664-5853

ANA/California
1250 Long Beach Ave, Ste. 323
Los Angeles, CA 90021
(213) 486-6555

Colorado Nurses Association
5453 East Evans Place
Denver, CO 80222
(303) 757-7483

Connecticut Nurses Association
Meritech Business Park
377 Research Parkway,
Suite 2D
Meriden, Connecticut 06450
(203)238-1207

Delaware Nurses
Association
2634 Capitol Trail,
Suite A
Newark, Delaware 19711
(302) 368-2333

District of Columbia
Nurses Association
5100 Wisconsin Avenue,
N.W. Suite 306
Washington, D.C. 20016
(202) 244-2705

Florida Nurses
Association
P.O. Box 536985
Orlando, FL 32853-6985
(407) 896-3261

Georgia Nurses Association
1362 West Peachtree Street NW
Atlanta, GA 30309
(404) 876-4624

Guam Nurses Association
P.O. Box CG
Agana, GU 96910
(011-671) 477-NURS

Hawaii Nurses Association
677 Ala Moana Blvd,
Suite 301
Honolulu, HI 96813
(808) 521-8361

Idaho Nurses Association
200 North 4th Street,
Suite 20
Boise, ID 83702-6001
(208) 345-0500

Illinois Nurses Association
300 South Wacker Drive
Suite 2200
Chicago, IL 60606
(312) 360-2300

Indiana State Nurses
Association
2915 North High School
Road
Indianapolis, IN 46224
(317) 299-4575

Iowa Nurses Association
150 42nd St., Ste. 471
Des Moines, IA 50266
(515) 225-0495

Kansas State Nurses
Association
700 S.W. Jackson, Suite 601
Topeka, KS 66603
(913) 233-8638

Kentucky Nurses Association
1400 South First Street
PO Box 2616
Louisville, KY 40201
(502) 637-2546

Louisiana State Nurses Association
712 Transcontinental Drive
Metaire, LA 70001
(504) 889-1030

Maine State Nurses Association
P.O. Box 2240
295 Water St.
Augusta, ME 04338-2240
(207) 622-1057

Maryland Nurses
Association
849 International Dr.
Airport Square 21, Ste. 255
Linthicum, MD 21090
(410) 859-3000

Massachusetts Nurses
Association
340 Turnpike Street
Canton, MA 02021
(617) 821-4625

Minnesota Nurses Association
1295 Bandana Boulevard
North, Suite 140
Saint Paul, MN
55108-5115
(612) 646-4807

Missouri Nurses Association
1904 Bubba Lane
Box 105228
Jefferson City, MO 65110
(314) 636-4623

Nebraska Nurses Association
1430 South St., Ste. 202
Lincoln, NE 68502-2446
(402) 475-3859

New Hampshire
Nurses Association
48 West Street
Concord, NH 03301-3595
(603) 225-3783

New Mexico Nurses
Association
909 Virginia NE, Ste. 101
Albuquerque, N M 87108
(505) 268-7744

Michigan Nurses
Association
2310 Jolly Oak Rd.
Okemos, MI 48864-4599
(517) 349-5640

Mississippi Nurses
Association
135 Bounds Street,
Suite 100
Jackson, MS 39206
(601) 982-9182

Montana Nurses Association
104 Broadway, Suite G-2
P.O. Box 5718
Helena, MT 59601
(406) 442-6710

Nevada Nurses Association
3660 Baker Lane, Suite 104
Reno, NV 89509
(702) 825-3555

New Jersey State
Nurses Association
320 West State Street
Trenton, N J 08618-5780
(609) 392-4884

New York State
Nurses Association
46 Cornell Rd.
Latham, NY 12110
(518) 782-9400

North Carolina
Nurses Association
Box 12025
103 Enterprise Street
Raleigh, NC  27605
(919) 821-4250

North Dakota State
Nurses Association
549 Airport Rd.
Bismark, ND  58504-6107
(701) 223-1385

Ohio Nurses Association
4000 East Main Street
Columbus, OH  43213-2983
(614) 237-5414

Oklahoma Nurses
Association
6414 North Santa Fe, Ste. A
Oklahoma City, OK  73116
(405) 840-3476

Oregon Nurses Association
9600 S.W. Oak, Suite 550
Portland, OR  97223
(503) 293-0011

Pennsylvania Nurses
Association
2578 Interstate Drive
P.O. Box 68525
Harrisburg, PA 17106-8525
(717) 657-1222

Rhode Island State
Nurses Association
550 South Water St.,
Unit 540B
Providence, RI  02903-4344
(401) 421-9703

South Carolina Nurses
Association
1821 Gadsden Street
Columbia, SC  29201
(803) 252-4781

South Dakota Nurses
Association
1505 South Minnesota Ave.,
Suite # 3
Sioux Falls, South Dakota
57105
(605) 338-1401

Tennessee Nurses
Association
545 Mainstream Drive
Suite 405
Nashville, TN  37228-1201
(615) 254-0350

Texas Nurses Association
7600 Burnet Rd.
Suite 440
Austin, TX  78757-1292
(512) 452-0645

Vermont State
Nurses Association
#26 Champlain Mill
1 Main St.
Winooski, VT  05404-2230
(802) 655-7123

Virginia Nurses Association
7113 Three Chopt Rd., Ste 204
Richmond, VA  23226
(804) 282-1808 or 282-2373

West Virginia Nurses
Association
2003 Quarrier St.
Charleston, WV  25311-4911
(304) 342-1169

Wyoming Nurses Association
Majestic Building, Room 305
1603 Capitol Avenue
Cheyenne, WY 82001
(307) 635-3955

Utah Nurses Association
455 East 400 South, #402
Salt Lake City, Utah 84111
(801) 322-3439

Virgin Islands Nurses
Association
P.O. Box 583
Christiansted
Saint Croix, Virgin Islands,
United States  00821
(809) 778-8328

Washington State Nurses Association
2505 Second Avenue, Suite 500
Seattle, WA  98121
(206) 443-9762

Wisconsin Nurses
Association
6117 Monona Drive
Madison, WI 53716
(608) 221-0383

# NURSES ORGANIZATIONS

American Nephrology Nurses
Association
Box 56
N Woodbury Road
Pitman, NJ 08071

American Association
of Nurse Anesthetists
222 S. Prospect Ave.
Park Ridge, IL 60068-4001

American Holistic
Nurses' Association
4101 Lake Boon Trail
Ste. 201
Raleigh, NC 27607

American Organization of
Nurse Executives
One N. Franklin
Chicago, IL 60606

Association of Operating
Room Nurses
2170 S. Parker Rd., Ste. 300
Denver, CO 80231

Association of
Rehabilitation Nurses
4700 W. Lake Dr.
1701 Lake Avenue
Glenview, IL 60025-1405

American Association of
Critical Care Nurses
101 Columbia
Aliso Viejo, CA 92656

American College
of Nurse Midwives
Suite 1000
1522 K Street NW
Washington, DC 20005

American Nurses
Association,
600 Maryland Ave.
Suite 100 W
Washington, DC 20024

Association for Practitioners
in Infection Control
23341 N. Milwaukee Avenue
Half Day, IL 60069

Association of Pediatric
Oncology Nurses
11512 Alleringie Parkway
Richmond, VA 23235

Association of Women's
Health, Obstetric and
Neonatal Nurses
700 14th St., NW, Ste 600
Washington, DC 20005-2006

National Organization for
the Advancement of Associate
Degree
11250 Roger Bacon Dr., Ste 8
Reston, VA  22090-5202

International Association
for Enterostomal Therapy
1701 Lake Avenue
Glenview, IL 60025

North American Nursing
Diagnosis Association
1211 Locust St.
Philadelphia, PA  19107

National Black Nurses
Association, Inc.
1511 K St.
Washington, DC  20005

National Association for
Men in Nursing
437 Twin Bay Dr.
Pensacola, FL  32534-1350

National Student Nurses
Association
Suite 1325
555 E. 57th Street
New York, NY 10019

Emergency Nurses Associa-
tion
230 E. Ohio
6th Floor
Chicago, IL 60611

International Council of
Nurses
3 Place Jean-Marteau
CH-1201
Geneva, Switzerland

National Association of
Pediatric Nurse Associates
and Practitioners
1101 Kings Highway N.
No. 206
Cherry Hill, NJ 08034-1912

National League for  Nursing
350 Hudson St.
New York, NY 10014

National  Nurses Society on
Addictions
5700 Old Orchard Rd.
1st Floor
Skokie, IL  60077

Nurses Christian Fellowship
PO Box 7895
Madison, WI 53707-7895

Oncology Nursing Society
501 Holiday Dr.
Pittsburgh, PA 15220

National Association of
Neonatal Nurses
1304 Southpoint Blvd.
Ste. 280
Petaluma, LA 94954

American Licensed Practical
Nurses Association
1090 Vermont Ave., NW
Ste. 1200
Washington, DC 20005

Sigma Theta Tau
National Honor
Society of Nursing
500 W. North St.
Indianapolis, IN 46202

World Health
Organization
Avenue Appia 1211
Geneva 27, Switzerland

# RESOURCES FOR MATERNAL
# CARE NURSES

## AIDS

AIDS MEDICAL FOUNDATION
10 EAST 13TH Street
Suite  LD
New York, NY   10003

## BREAST FEEDING

LaLeche International, Inc.
9616 Minneapolis Avenue
Franklin Park, IL 60123

## CHILDBIRTH INFORMATION

American Academy of
Husband-Coached Childbirth
P.O. Box 5224
Sherman Oaks, CA 91413

American College of Home Obstetrics
P.O. Box 508
Oak Park, IL 60303

American Society of Childbirth Educators
P.O. Box 2282
Sedona, AZ  86339

American Society for
Psychoprophylaxis in Obstetrics
1200 19th St., N.W., Ste 300
Washington, DC 20036-2412


C/SEC
22 Forest Rd.
Framingham, MA 01701


Childbirth Education Foundation
P.O. Box 5
Richboro, PA 18954


Childbirth Without Pain Education Association
20134 Snowden
Detroit, MI 48235


Informed Homebirth/Informed Birth and Parenting
P.O. Box 3675
Ann Arbor, MI 48106


Maternity Center Association, Inc.
48 East 92nd Street
New York, New York 10028


Read Natural Childbirth Foundation
P.O. Box 150956
San Rafael, CA 94915

## FAMILY PLANNING

Planned Parenthood Federation of America, Inc.
810 - 7th Ave.
New York, NY 10019

National Family Planning and Reproductive
Health Association
122 C. St., N.W., Ste 380
Washington, DC 20007

## FERTILITY STUDIES

American Fertility Foundation
1231 Magnolia Ave., Ste. 201
Birmingham, AL 35205

American Society for Reproductive Medicine
1209 Montgomery Highway
Birmingham, AL 35216-2809

Fertility Research Foundation
877 Park Ave.
New York, NY 10021

## GENETIC COUNSELING

American Board of Genetic Counseling
9650 Rockville Pike
Bethesda, MD  20814-3998

National Society of Genetic Counselors
233 Canterbury Dr.
Wallingford, PA  19086

## PARENTING AND CONCERNS

Family Therapy Sect. of the National Council
on Family Relations
3989 Central Ave., N.E., No. 550
Minneapolis, MN  55421

Department of Health, Education, and Welfare
US Children's Bureau Office of Child Development
P.O. Box 1182
Washington, DC 20013

Healthy Mothers, Healthy Babies
409 - 12th St., S.W., Room 309
Washington, DC  20024

National Committee to Prevent Child  Abuse
332 S. Michigan Ave., Ste. 1600
Chicago, IL 60604

United Grief Support
7600 Central Ave.
Philadelphia, PA  19111-2499

Parents  Anonymous
675 W. Foothill Blvd., Ste. 220
Claremont, CA  91711-3416

Parents Reaching Out
PO Box 121806
Nashville, TN  37212-1806

Parents Without Partners
401 N. Michigan Ave.
Chicago, IL  60611-4267

Single Mothers by Choice
PO Box 1642, Grace Square Station
New York, NY  10028

## PROFESSIONAL ORGANIZATIONS

American Foundation for Maternal and Child Health
439 E. 51st, 4th Floor
New York, NY  10022

American College of Nurse-Midwives
1522 K St, NW, Suite 1000
Washington, DC 20005

American College of Obstetricians and  Gynecologists
409 - 12th St., S.W.
Washington, DC 20024

Maternity Center Association, Inc.
48 E 92nd Street
New York, NY 10028

## PUBLIC HEALTH ORGANIZATIONS

American Public Health Association
1015 15th Street, NW
Washington, DC 20005

American Red Cross
430 17th St., N.W.
Washington, DC 20006

Centers for Disease Control
1600 Clifton Rd., N.E.
Atlanta, GA 30333

National Institute of Child Health and Human
Development
National Institutes of Health
9000 Rockville Pike, Bldg. 31
Room 2432
Bethesda, MD 20892

## SEX EDUCATION AND THERAPY

American Association of Sex Educators,
Counselors and Therapists
435 N. Michigan Ave., Ste. 1717
Chicago, IL  60611

Council for Sex Information and Education
2272 Colorado Blvd., No. 1228
Los Angeles, CA  90041

## SEXUALLY-TRANSMITTED DISEASES

American Foundation for Prevention
of Venereal Disease
799 Broadway, Ste. 638
New York, NY 10003


American Social Health Association
P.O. Box 13827
Research Triangle Park, NC 27709


Herpes Resource Center
American Social Health Association
P. O. Box 13827
Research Triangle Park, NC 27709

# APPENDIX A

# APPENDIX A

AWHONN Standards & Guidelines
Table of Contents. . . . . . . . . . . . . . . . . . . 279
Selected Obstetric AWHONN Guidelines . . . . . . 281
AWHONN PDMS Phone Number . . . . . . . . . 290
AWHONN On-Line Address . . . . . . . . . . . 290

# AWHONN Standards & Guidelines

## Table of Contents

Acknowledgments . . . . . . . . . . . . . . . . . . . iii

Preface . . . . . . . . . . . . . . . . . . . . . . . . V

Introduction to the Fifth Edition . . . . . . . . . . . ix

**SECTION I**

Standards of Care . . . . . . . . . . . . . . . . . . . 1

Standards of Professional Performance . . . . . . . . 3

**SECTION II**

Introduction to the Guidelines . . . . . . . . . . . . 9

**General Women's Health**

Guideline for a Nursing Health Assessment
in Mid-Life Women . . . . . . . . . . . . . . . . . . 10

**Perinatal and Newborn Health**

Guideline for Health Education and Perinatal
and Newborn Nursing . . . . . . . . . . . . . . . 12

**Guideline for Planning Family-Centered
Care to Meet the Needs of the Mother
and Baby** . . . . . . . . . . . . . . . . . . . **14**

**Guideline for the Care of the Healthy
Newborn** . . . . . . . . . . . . . . . . . . . . **16**

Guideline for Breastfeeding Support . . . . . . . . 18

Guideline for Providing Care to the Family
Experiencing Perinatal Loss and Fetal Death . . . 20

## Acute Care

Guideline for Resuscitation of the Pregnant Woman and the Newborn . . . . . . . . . . . . . . . . . . 23

Guideline for Identifying the Appropriate Care Site for Pregnant Women Requiring Critical Care . . . 25

Guideline for Perioperative and Perianalgesia/Anesthesia Care of the Pregnant Woman . . . . . . . . . . . . . . . . . . . . . . . . 28

## Community/Home Care

Guideline for Home Care of Women and Newborns . . . . . . . . . . . . . . . . . . . . . . 36

## Administration

Guideline for Management of Staffing Resources . . . . . . . . . . . . . . . . . . . . . . . 38

Glossary . . . . . . . . . . . . . . . . . . . . . . . . 43

# Guideline for Planning Family-Centered Care to Meet the Needs of the Mother and Baby

## PURPOSE

The purpose of family-centered perinatal care is to support the role of women in promoting their own health and well-being and that of their children and families. This form of care provides a structure for a collaborative relationship between the perinatal care provider and the family in decision-making and planning. The family's individual needs and responsibilities are recognized. Family-centered care sets the tone for respect of diversity in family structure and cultural backgrounds. Caring for the mother and baby together (couplet care) is a unified approach that nurtures attachment in the new family.

## DEFINITION OF TERMS

*Family-centered perinatal care* is a model of care based on the philosophy that the physical, social, psychological, spiritual, and economic needs of the total family unit, however the family may be defined, should be integrated and considered collectively. It requires a collaborative relationship between the childbearing woman and her family and health care professionals.

*Mother-baby (couplet) care*, a critical component of the family-centered philosophy, reflects the family-centered perspective for assessment, planning, and delivery of care to women and newborns. The focus of mother-baby nursing care is teaching and role modeling, while providing bedside care to the mother and baby together.

## METHODOLOGY

1. The nurse uses the following methods to facilitate family-centered care:

   * Creates a supportive, safe, functional, and welcoming environment for women and their families

   * Recognizes women and their families as integral members of the health care team and encourages them to enter into decision-making and planning of care

   * Promotes the concept of pregnancy, labor, birth, and the postpartum period as a continuum and as a time of emotional, social and physical change

   * Provides childbirth education that promotes freedom of choice based on knowledge of options, individual preferences, priorities, and goals

   * Provides prenatal and parenting education that reflects the cultures of the families served and is based on their needs

   * Works in partnership with families, assisting but not directing them

   * Provides individualized, flexible care

   * Empowers and educates families for childbearing and parenting to promote positive, healthy families

* Respects cultural beliefs and values of women and their families

* Advocates nonseparation of the baby from the parents or support person(s)

* Encourages the other parent or support person(s) to be present, as the mother desires, and actively involved in labor and birth as well as with postpartum and newborn care

* Involves families in planning and evaluating care

2. A family-centered program includes the following elements:

* A family-centered mission and philosophy statement for ambulatory and inpatient programs of care

* Patient advisory groups that collaborate with professionals in developing and evaluating programs

* Care programs scheduled to be accessible to families

* Classes to prepare for childbirth and parenting, as well as parenting support groups

* Medical record documentation and a data management system that respect a woman's right to privacy

* Personnel practices that support staff in providing family-centered, culturally sensitive care

* Policies and staff that respect and support the decision made by women and their families

* Mother-baby nursing during the postpartum period

* Support, education, and counseling regarding lactation

* A comprehensive approach that links women and their babies and families with follow-up support services and health care providers in their community

* Support for families of babies with special medical and developmental needs, with emphasis on the family's role as primary caregiver

3.  In facilitating the unified plan for mother-baby (couplet) care, the nurse uses the following methods:

* Assesses the educational needs of the family and barriers to learning

* Performs neonatal assessment at the mother's bedside as an opportunity for the mother to learn about her baby's unique physical and behavioral characteristics

* Performs maternal assessment as an opportunity for the mother to learn about postpartum self-care and parenting

* Integrates the whole family into care of the mother and baby

* Provides lactation support for the breastfeeding mother that facilitates mother-infant contact both day and night

* Coordinates care to support the mother's and baby's unique response patterns

* Refers the family to community agencies and resources as appropriate

* Measures teaching outcomes to determine the new mother's understanding about care and feeding of her baby and about self-care

*This guideline was developed under the direction of the AWHONN Committee on Practice. The guideline suggests a general guideline for practice. Additional or different considerations or procedures may be warranted for particular patient settings. The best interest of an individual patient is always the touchstone of practice. The guideline is not intended to prescribe an exclusive course of action or to establish an obligatory standard of practice for legal, regulatory or other purposes.*

## BIBLIOGRAPHY

Karen, R. (1997). *Becoming attached: Unfolding the mystery of the infant-mother bond and its impact on later life.* New York: Oxford University Press.

Klaus, M.H., Kennell, J.H., & Klaus, P.H. (1995). *Bonding: Building the foundations of secure attachment and independence.* Reading, MA: Addison-Wesley.

Phillips, C.R. (1996). *Family-centered maternity and newborn care: A basic text.* St. Louis, MO: Mosby-Year Book.

Phillips, C.R. (1994). *Family-centered maternity care.* Minneapolis, MN: International Childbirth Education Association.

Symanski, M.E. (1992). Maternal-infant bonding: Practice issues for the 1990's. *Journal of Nurse Midwifery, 37,* 67-73.

Tomlison, P.S., Bryan, A.A.M, & Esau, A.L. (1996). Family centered intrapartum care: Revising an old concept. *Journal of Obstetric, Gynecologic, and Neonatal Nursing, 25,* 331-337.

# Guideline for the Care of the Healthy Newborn

## PURPOSE

Nurses provide care for healthy newborns in a variety of settings. Regardless of the setting, the principles of care are similar. Nurses coordinate or participate directly in the care of newborns and monitor their growth and development from birth to follow-up care.

## DEFINITION OF TERMS

*Newborn* refers to an infant from birth to 28 days of life. The *healthy newborn* is an individual who is expected to complete the transition to extrauterine life without complications.

*Stabilization* usually occurs during the first 6 to 12 hours after birth. During this period, the infant makes the transition to extrauterine life, a process that involves behavioral changes and changes in all body systems, with emphasis on cardiorespiratory, metabolic, and endocrine systems and the central nervous system.

## METHODOLOGY

The nurse provides the following care to the healthy newborn, much of which is delineated in the *Guidelines for Perinatal Care* (1997):

* Conducts the initial assessment of the infant, which may include

  * Proper identification of the newborn

  * Physical assessments and review of the maternal history within 2 hours of birth to determine the newborn's risk or risk factors

* Provides prophylactic eye care within 1 hour of birth and other medications as indicated during stabilization

* Develops a plan of care for the newborn, which includes appropriate observations during stabilization and for the remainder of the time the newborn is under the nurse's care

* Makes anticipatory observations of the newborn in the stabilization period. Observations may include but are not limited to monitoring of temperature, heart rate, type of respiration and respiratory rate, skin color, adequacy of peripheral circulation, level of consciousness, tone, and activity

* Records observations of the newborn at least every 30 minutes until the newborn's condition has remained stable for 2 hours

* Documents that the primary health care provider of the healthy newborn conducts a physical examination no later than 24 hours after birth and within 24 hours before discharge

* Documents the newborn's weight at least daily

* Implements emergency measures, including resuscitation, when necessary, using the guidelines of programs such as the Neonatal Resuscitation Program of the American Heart Association and American Academy of Pediatrics Neonatal Resuscitation Program Steering Committee (1995)

* Observes parent-infant interactions, including the mother's ability to talk to the newborn, explore the newborn's physical appearance, and identify individual characteristics. Observes the newborn's behavior and reciprocity, which may include the ability to establish eye contact with the mother in the en face position. These activities suggest mother-infant attachment

* Teaches the parent(s) activities of daily living for the newborn, which may include but are not limited to bathing, cord care, and circumcision care; information regarding newborn crying characteristics, elimination, and sleep patterns; and the importance of handwashing

* Verifies before discharge that state or Canadian province screening tests for the newborn, as required by law, have been completed, and that parents are aware of the need for any follow-up testing

* Identifies with parent(s) the appropriate facility for follow-up care and emergency procedures. Addresses the need for regular appointments and how to obtain them

* Informs the parent(s) of the importance of immunizations, the recommended schedule for immunizations, and where they can be obtained

* Identifies mothers whose high-risk behaviors may affect the health of their infants and assists in making referrals

\* Evaluates the home environment for the following when practice is based in the community: newborn safety, including water and ambient air temperature; crib safety; storage of milk; and use of a car seat

*This guideline was developed under the direction of the AWHONN Committee on Practice. The guideline suggests a general guideline for practice. Additional or different considerations or procedures may be warranted for particular patient settings. The best interest of an individual patient is always the touchstone of practice. The guideline is not intended to prescribe an exclusive course of action or to establish an obligatory standard of practice for legal, regulatory or other purposes.*

## REFERENCES

American Academy of Pediatrics & American College of Obstetricians and Gynecologists. (1997). *Guidelines for perinatal care* (4th ed.). Elk Grove Village, IL: Author.

American Heart Association & American Academy of Pediatrics Neonatal Resuscitation Program Steering Committee. (1995). *Textbook of neonatal resuscitation.* Dallas, TX: Author

*To order the AWHONN Standards and Guidelines for Professional Nursing Practice in the Care of Women and Newborns, 5th Edition, contact AWHONN via:*

1.  PDMS Phone Number:  1 (800) 354-2268
2.  On-Line:  www.awhonn.org

# APPENDIX B: CERVICAL DILATATION

# CERVICAL DILATATION

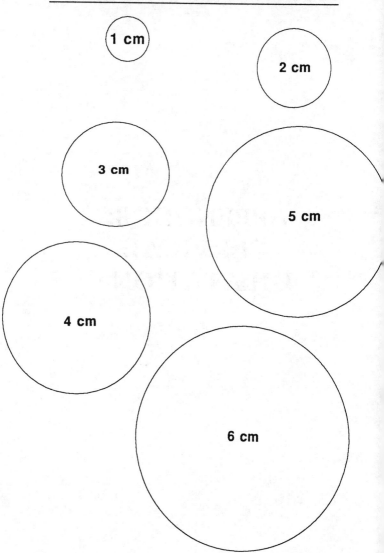

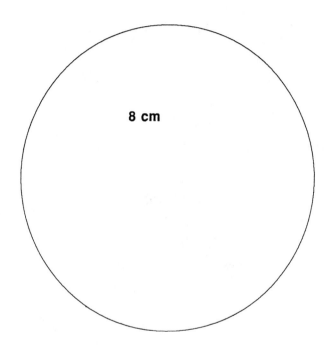

8 cm

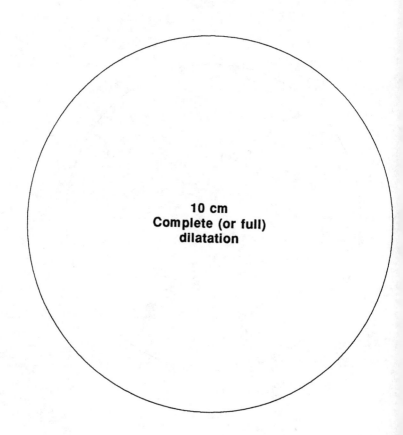

**10 cm**
**Complete (or full)**
**dilatation**

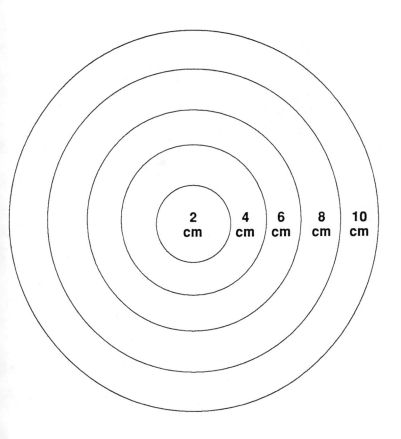

# Index

24 hour clock, 193

**A**

Abbreviations, 184-191

Abruptio Placentae, 134

Abstinence, 163

Acne, 156

Adenoma, 157

Alba, 110

Alcohol, 30, 107, 230

Alkaline phosphatase, 179

Aloe, 197

Amenhorrea, 155, 158

Amniocentesis, 177-178

Anemia, 34, 47, 162

Ankle edema, 39

Assessment, 234

Atropine, 197

Avocadoes, 118

**B**

Backache, 107

Barbiturates, 197, 230

Barriers to Communication, 238

Beef, 117

Bilirubin, 178-179

Direct, 181

Total, 181

Biographical data, 22

Biographical information, 22, 29

Bleeding, 38-39

Bloating, 108

Blood pressure
Neonatal, 183

Blood smear, 178

Bloody show, 112

Boards of Nursing, 250

Bradycardia, 183

Breads, 117

Breakthrough bleeding, 155

Breast cancer, 157

Breast changes, 105

Breast engorgement, 111

Breastfeeding, 149

Breasts, 146

Breathing techniques, 114

Burst of energy, 113

Butter, 118

**C**

Caffeine, 130

Calcium, 128-130

Carbohydrates
 Complex, 122
 Simple, 122

Carbohydrates (complex), 122

Carbon monoxide, 230

Cardiac disease, 158

Cereal, 117

Cervical cap, 160

Cervical changes, 112

Charting, 239, 241

Cheese, 117

Chills, 38-39

Chloasma, 107

Chloral hydrate, 197

Chloramphenicol, 197

Cholestatic jaundice, 157

Chorionic villus sampling, 178

Clotting factors
 Neonatal, 179

Cocaine, 230

Collaboration, 13

Collegiality, 12

Complications, 47

Complications of pregnancy, 134

Condom, 160

Constipation, 109

Contraception, 152, 158
 Barrier Methods, 160
 Oral, 155

Contraceptives
 Biphasic, 153
 Monophasic, 153
 Triphasic, 153

Contraction stress test, 178

Contractions, 113-115
 Braxton-Hicks, 109, 112

Copper, 129-130

Cottage cheese, 117

Cramping
 Abdominal, 141

Cramps
 Leg, 39, 106

Cream, 118

Cream cheese, 118

Creatinine clearance, 179

Creatinine level, 178

Cullen's signs, 141

Current medical history, 25

Cyclophosphamide, 197

**D**

Dairy products, 117

Depo-Provera, 197

Developmental history, 26

Diabetes, 157

Diabetes mellitus, 34

Diaphragm, 160

Diarrhea, 38-39, 151

Diazepam, 197

Dicumarol, 197

Diethylstilbestrol, 197

Dihydrotachysterol, 197

Dilatation, 113-115

Dizziness, 39

Documentation, 239

Doppler auscultation, 42

Drug use, 31
    Over-the-counter, 32

Drugs
    Illegal, 107

Dysmenhorrea, 161

Dyspareunia, 107

**E**

Eclampsia, 34, 139

Ectopic pregnancy, 140, 155, 162

Edema, 42, 108, 140, 154
    Ankle, 39
    Generalized, 39

Education, 11

Effacement, 113-115

Effleurage, 114

Eggs, 117

Elimination, 146-147

Endometrium, 160

Epigastric pain, 39

Episiotomy, 111, 149

Epistaxis, 37, 106

Ergot, 197

Estimated date of delivery (EDD), 40

Estrogen, 149, 152-153

Ethics, 12

Ethinyl estradiol, 197

Evaluation, 236

Exercise, 30, 39

# F

Faintness, 38

Fallopian tube, 160

Family dynamics, 39

Fatigue, 39, 106

Fats, 118, 128

FDA Pregnancy Categories, 199

Fertilization, 160

Fetal heart rate, 42

Fetal heartbeat, 115

Fetal movement, 40, 43

Fetal movements, 38

Fetal position, 115

Fetal presentation, 43

Fetoscope auscultation, 42

Fever, 38-39

Fibrinogen, 178, 181

Fibroadenomas, 155

First trimester, 37, 105

    Danger signs, 38

    Discomforts, 37

    Self-care, 37

Fish, 117

Flagyl, 197

Flatulence, 108

Folate, 129

Folate indices, 176

Folic acid, 126

Foods

    Calcium-rich, 132

    Fast, 131

    High-sodium, 132

    Iron-rich, 133

    Potassium-rich, 131

    Tyramine, 133

    Vitamin-K rich, 132

Fruits and vegetables, 118

Fundal height, 43

Fundus, 110

# G

Gastrointestinal distress, 38

Genetic counseling, 35

Genital tract anomaly, 34

Gingivitis, 37-39

Gold, 197

Gonorrhea, 162

Grain products, 117

Green vegetables, 118

Gynecologic history, 24

# H

Head-to-Toe Systems Assessment, 239
Headache, 39, 154
Headaches, 106, 156
Height and weight chart, 46
    Women, 46
HELLP, 137
HELLP Syndrome, 139
Hemoglobin, 43
Hemorrhoids, 109, 111, 143
Heroin, 197
Heroine, 230
High-sodium foods, 132
Hirsutism, 155
History of abuse, 28
History of illness, 23
Homan's sign, 42
Human immuno-deficiency virus, 156
Human immuno-deficiency virus (HIV), 177
Hydramnios, 47
Hyperemesis gravidarum, 136

Hyperglycemia, 47
Hypermenorrhea, 155
Hypertension, 47, 154, 157
Hypomenhorrea, 154
Hypomenorrhea, 155
Hypovolemic shock, 141

# I

Indomethacin, 197
Infant care
    Bathing, 150
    Diapering, 150
    Feeding, 149
Infant-care, 149
Initial interview, 21
Insomnia, 39, 109
Intervention, 235
Involution, 110
Iron, 122, 129
Iron indices, 176
Isoniazid, 197

# J

Job interview, 249

# K

Kegel exercises, 143

Kegel's exercises, 108, 110

**L**

Labor
    False, 39
    Preterm, 39
Labor, stages of , 109
Laboratory findings
    Pregnancy, 175
Laboratory tests
    Hematocrit, 43
Laboratory values
    Blood sugar/glucose, 170
    Cardiovascular determinations, 171
    Chest x-ray studies, 172
    Hematologic, 167
    Hepatic values, 172
    Mineral/Vitamin concentrations, 170
    Neonatal, 179
    Renal values, 173
    Serum proteins, 170
Lactation, 112, 146
Legumes, 117
Lethargy, 151

Letting-go phase, 142
Leukorrhea, 37, 105
Lightening, 112
Lithium, 197
Lithium carbonate, 230
Liver disease, 158
Liver function tests, 177
Lochia, 110

**M**

Magnesium sulfate, 230
Malnutrition, 105
Malpractice
    Prevention of, 243
Maternal comfort, 143
    Abdominal, 144
    Breast, 144
    Perineal, 143
    Rest measures, 145
    Sleep measures, 145
Maternal self-care, 147
    Afterpains, 148
    Breasts, 147
    Elimination, 148
    Exercise, 148
    Immunizations, 149
    Nutrition, 148

Perineal, 147

Rest, 148

Maternal serum alpha-
  fetoprotein (MSAF),
  43

Meat Group, 117

Medical history

  Family, 29

  Partner's, 32

  Partner's family, 32

  Past, 25

Melasma, 154, 156

Membranes

  Rupture of, 38-39, 113

Menstrual cycles, 164

Meprobamate, 197

Methamphetamine, 230

Methergine
  (methylergonovine),
  230

Methotrexate, 197

Milk, 117

Monolial vaginitis, 155

Morning sickness, 105

Multigravida, 142

Multiparity, 163

Multiparous, 161

Muscular comfort, 144

**N**

NANDA Nursing Diag-
  noses, 234

Nasal stuffiness, 37, 106

Nausea, 105, 154

Neuromuscular distress,
  38

Niacin, 127

Nonstress test, 178

Nulliparous, 156

Nurses organizations, 266

Nursing process, 233

Nutrient supplementa-
  tion, 129

Nutrition, 37-39, 47, 146

Nutritional assessment,
  36

Nuts, 117-118

**O**

Occupational history, 29,
  32

Oil, 118

Ova, 160, 162

Ovarian cysts, 155-156

**P**

Pain, 113-115

    After pains, 110

Palpitations, 38

Pap smear, 160

Past pregnancy history, 24

Pasta, 117

Peanut butter, 117

Pelvic inflammatory disease (PID), 155, 161

Percutaneous umbilical blood sampling, 178

Performance appraisal, 11

Perineum, 145

Phenothiazines, 197

Phenylbutazone, 197

Phosphatidylglycerol, 178

Phosphorus, 127

Physical assessment

    Neonate, 85

Physiologic well-being, 145

Placenta, 149

Placenta previa, 135

Planning/outcome criteria, 235

Platelets, 175, 178

Pork, 117

Postpartum depression, 111

Postpartum psychosis, 111

Potassium, 127

Potassium-rich foods, 131

Poultry, 117

Preeclampsia, 34

    Mild, 138

    Severe, 138

Pregnancy weight gain, 43

Pregnancy-induced hypertension, 137

Prenatal risk factors, 42

Primigravida, 142

Progestin, 152-153

Protein, 121

Prothrombin, 178

Psychological history, 26

Psychosocial history, 42

Psychosocial responses, 38

Puerperium, 141, 151

Pulmonary embolism, 158

Pyrosis, 108

## Q
Quality of care, 10
Quickening, 43
Quinine, 197

## R
Recommended daily allowances
  Pregnant and lactating women, 120
Recommended daily allowances
  Women, 119
Relaxation techniques, 114
Renal plasma flow, 175
Research, 13
Reserpine, 197
Resource utilization, 15
Resources, 269
Resume, 247
Rh negative mother, 47
RhoGAM, 149
Rice, 117
Rubella, 149
Rubra, 110

## S
Second trimester, 38, 107
  Danger signs, 38
  Discomforts, 38
  Self-care, 38
Seeds, 117
Senna, 197
Serous, 110
Serum folate, 176
Serum uric acid, 175
Sexual activity, 40, 149
Sexual history, 25
Sexuality, 39
Sexually-transmitted disease (STD), 156, 159, 160
Sickle cell disease, 34
Sickle cell hemoglobinopathy, 157
Signs of Labor
  Premonitory, 112
Skin changes, 38
Sleep, 30
Smoking, 107
Sodium, 127
Sperm, 160
Spermicides, 159

Sponge, 160

Standards of Care, 5

    Assessment, 7

    Diagnosis, 7

    Evaluation, 9

    Implementation, 9

    Outcome identification, 8

    Planning, 8

Standards of Clinical Nursing Practice, 5

Standards of Professional Performance, 6

Station, 115

Streptomycin, 230

Striae gravidarum, 107

Sulfonamides, 197

Syphilis, 47

**T**

Tachycardia, 177, 183

Taking-hold phase, 142

Taking-in phase, 142

Tampons, 147

Temperature, 150

Teratogens, 47

Tetracycline, 230

Thalidomide, 230

Third trimester, 39, 108

    Danger signs, 39

    Discomforts, 39

    Self-care, 39

Thrombocytopenia, 175

Thromboembolism, 157

Thrombophlebitis, 158

Thyroid function tests, 177

Toxic shock syndrome (TSS), 160

Tubal ligation, 162

**U**

Ultrasound, 178

Umbilical cord, 150

Urinalysis, 43, 182

Urinary frequency, 106, 109

Urinary retention, 110

Urinary tract infections, 160

Urination, 38

Urine acidifiers, 133

Uterine anomalies, 162

## V

Vagina, 149

Varicose veins, 106

Varicosities, 38

Vas deferens, 162

Vasectomy, 162

Vertigo, 106

Vital signs, 141

Vitamin A, 123

Vitamin B, 176

Vitamin B1 (Thiamin), 123

Vitamin B12 (Cobalamin), 124, 130

Vitamin B2 (Riboflavin), 123

Vitamin B6 (Pyridoxine), 124, 129

Vitamin C, 125, 129

Vitamin D, 125, 129

Vitamin E, 126

Vitamin K, 126

Vomiting, 38, 105

## W

Weight gain, 40

## Y

Yogurt, 117

## Z

Zinc, 128-130